CLINICAL
ULTRASOUND

CLINICAL ULTRASOUND

A HOW-TO GUIDE

EDITED BY

Tarina Lee Kang

University of Southern California
Department of Emergency Medicine
Los Angeles, CA, USA

John Bailitz

Emergency Ultrasound Division Director
Department of Emergency Medicine
Cook County Hospital (Stroger)
Associate Professor of Emergency Medicine
Rush University Medical School

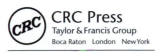

CRC Press
Taylor & Francis Group
Boca Raton London New York

CRC Press is an imprint of the
Taylor & Francis Group, an **informa** business

Contents

Preface

ABOUT THIS BOOK

- Provides a pocket-sized, practical "How-To Guide" for the busy clinician learning clinical ultrasound on the job.
- Written by experts in emergency medicine clinical ultrasound from across the United States.
- Chapter information is presented in the order of use: indications, image acquisition, image interpretation, integration of findings, and special considerations.
- Many truly outstanding ultrasound reference textbooks and more detailed handbooks already exist. We are indebted to these authors for their expertise and dedication. This book is intended as a supplemental, rapid, bedside tutorial for the clinical arena.
- Key references and websites at the end of the book provide opportunities for additional learning.

Introduction

Gavin Budhram MD, Tarina Lee Kang MD, John Bailitz MD

HISTORY OF CLINICAL ULTRASOUND (CUS)

- 1950s: Medical ultrasound not widely utilized because patients were required to be submerged in water during the study.
- 1970s: More advanced ultrasound machines are developed for use in limited clinical settings.
- 1980s: Real-time ultrasound that generates an image without appreciable delay between signal generation and image display is developed.
- Additional technological improvements result in smaller, faster, and more portable machines. Multi-frequency probes and color Doppler is developed. Initial feasibility and accuracy studies are completed for multiple new clinical applications.
- 2001 and 2008: The American College of Emergency Physicians (ACEP) publishes their position papers defining the clinical indications and training curricula for emergency CUS.
- 2000s: More advanced CUS applications proposed. Initial outcomes trials are conducted in the United States.
- 2011: More than twenty-one different medical specialties are now utilizing CUS to improve patient care.

BENEFITS OF CUS

- Answers common clinical questions immediately at the bedside.
- Expedites initiation of care with greater diagnostic confidence.
- Provides vital initial hemodynamic information followed by response to therapy for unstable patients.
- Helpful when the history is unobtainable or the physical exam is difficult.
- Incurs no risk to the patient or healthcare provider.
- Faster and less expensive than other imaging studies.
- Portable and effective even in resource-limited environments.
- Requires considerable initial and ongoing training, yet may be utilized rapidly with appropriate supervision.

DIAGNOSTIC CONSIDERATIONS

- The CUS clinician is both the operator and the interpreter of the focused bedside imaging study. Information is obtained and interpreted in real time without delays for transport and outside interpretation.
- CUS answers binary clinical questions by readily identifying normal and pathologic findings relevant to a clinician's particular scope of practice.
- CUS provides a useful adjunct to patient care though is not a replacement for more comprehensive imaging studies.

PHYSICS AND ARTIFACTS

- Sound characteristics: Human hearing is in the range of 20–20,000 Hertz (cycles per second). Ultrasound is greater than 20 KHz. Diagnostic ultrasound is greater than 1,000,000 Hz (1 MHz).
- Piezoelectric effect: Crystals with piezoelectric (pressure-electricity) properties vibrate in response to an applied electrical charge, producing ultrasound waves that are emitted into the patient's body. Sound waves propagate through the body at a constant speed, reflect off anatomical structures, and finally return to the probe. Crystals then vibrate in response to returning sound waves, producing an electrical signal that is sent to the processor.
- Probes listen more than talk: Ultrasound transducers "transmit" sound approximately 1% of the time and "receive" sound 99% of the time.
- Two-dimensional grayscale ultrasound images are created based on the strength of returning sound wave (brightness of the pixel on the US screen), and round trip time (depth of the pixel in the body on the US screen).
- Sound transmission is influenced by density and stiffness of tissue.
    - Density: High density tissue (liver, spleen, water) transmits sound better than lower density tissue (air).
    - Stiffness: Flexible tissue (liver, spleen) transmits sound better than stiff tissue (bone).
- Sound waves behave in different ways depending on the tissue.
    - Reflection: A portion of the sound energy is reflected back to transducer when a tissue plane is struck. An ultrasound machine uses this information to generate an image.
    - Attenuation: A portion of the sound energy is lost each time a wave strikes successively deeper tissue layers. Hence, the image appears relatively darker in the deeper field.
    - Scatter: Ultrasound beams scatter when striking an interface smaller than the sound beam. The beam does not return to the transducer and this information is lost. This creates a hyperechoic (bright white) air artifact with mixed echogenicity (dirty gray) shadows.
    - Refraction: The sound beam may be redirected if entering a tissue with a different propagation speed. This creates, for instance, an anechoic edge artifact at the edge of the gallbladder.

- Absorption: A small portion of the sound energy is changed to heat energy and dissipates. This is the basis for the ALARA principle = As Low As Reasonably Achievable. For example, Doppler assessments of fetal heart rate are not routinely performed due to the risk of damage to the fetal heart from the sound energy.

ULTRASOUND ARTIFACTS

US artifacts must be understood in order to properly identify both normal and abnormal findings. Remember, the image viewed on the ultrasound screen is only a sonographic representation of the tissue. Many of the classic artifacts are routinely seen in gallbladder CUS.

- Acoustic enhancement: Area deep to a fluid-filled anechoic cystic structure appears brighter than the surrounding tissue (*). This creates an "acoustic window" when imaging organs posterior to cystic structures. For example, the bladder creates an acoustic window through which to view an early intrauterine pregnancy on transabdominal ultrasound.

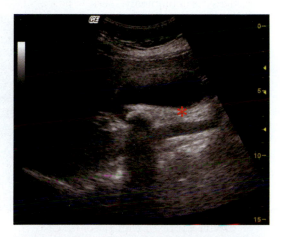

- Shadowing: Area deep to a highly reflective surface appears dark (*). This occurs when the sound beam cannot penetrate through tissue. For example, dense and stiff structures such as bone, gallstones, and kidney stones produce bright hyperechogenic structures with characteristic dark anechoic shadows. In contrast, low density bowel gas is a poorly reflective

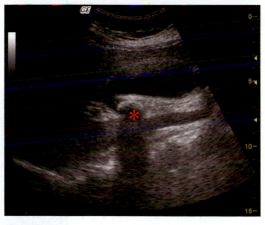

surface that scatters acoustic energy, creating poorly defined hyperechoic areas with characteristic "dirty" shadows of mixed echogenicity. These differences allow the clinician to distinguish between gallstones, and air in the duodenum next to the gallbladder.

- Mirroring: Mirror image of a structure is seen on the opposite side of a highly reflective surface. This occurs when sound bounces off the reflective surface before reaching the structure of interest and returning back to the probe. The ultrasound machine interprets the longer transit time as a second structure. This is commonly seen along the diaphragm (*). Absence of this "normal" artifact suggests the presence of a pleural effusion.

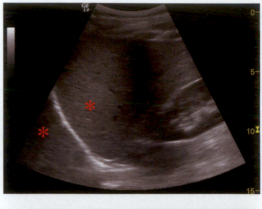

- Edge artifact: The areas lateral and deep to a cystic structure appear dark when sound is refracted off the sides. This may disappear when imaged in an orthogonal plane. This artifact is commonly found around the gallbladder and may be confused with gall-

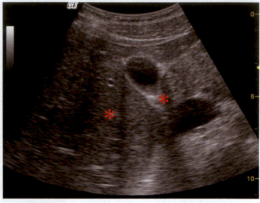

stones (*). Gallstones are hyperechogenic with anechoic shadows that move when the patient changes position.

- Side lobe artifact: Represents internal reflections inside of a cystic structure. This occurs when the ultrasound beam leaves the transducer, and although is still extremely narrow, has a small but measurable width. Beams originating at an angle to the main beam strike the sides of the cystic structure and are reflected off at different angles. These may disappear when imaged in an orthogonal plane. May be confused with "sludge" inside the gallbladder which exists in two planes in dependent areas.

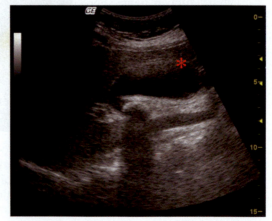

- Reverberation: Recurrent bright arcs at equidistant spacing from two highly reflective surfaces.

This occurs when sound waves bounce repeatedly between two reflective surfaces before returning to the probe. It is often seen at the anterior aspect of the urinary bladder, or extending downward from the pleural interface of the lung (*). May disappear when imaged in an orthogonal plane and when reducing the gain.

TRANSDUCERS, KNOBOLOGY, AND ORIENTATION

- Ultrasound transducers (probes) vary with regard to frequency, footprint, and crystal array type.
- Frequency: Most probes are designed to work over a range of frequencies. Higher frequency probes have better resolution but less depth of penetration.
  - Lower frequency transducers (1–5 MHz) penetrate deeper tissues at the expense of image quality. This frequency is generally better suited for deep cardiac imaging.
  - Medium frequency transducers (3–8 MHz) have medium penetration and image quality. This frequency is generally better suited for abdominal imaging.
  - High frequency transducers (5–10 MHz) have high resolution but sacrifice depth penetration. This frequency is generally better suited for vascular or soft tissue imaging.
- Footprint: The size of the membrane overlying the crystal array.
  - Cardiac transducers have smaller footprints to fit between intercostal spaces.
  - Abdominal transducers have large, rounded footprints to cover more surface area at greater depths.
- Arrays: Represent the arrangement of piezoelectric crystals under the footprint.
  - Linear array: Crystals are arranged in a straight line and transmit ultrasound beams in a perpendicular direction. Image is rectangular shaped.
  - Convex (curvilinear) array: Crystals are arranged in a convex arc under a rounded footprint and transmit ultrasound beams in a fan-shaped distribution. Image is wedge shaped.

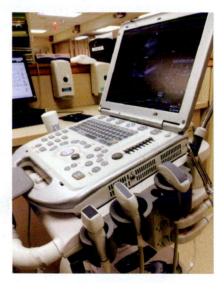

  - Phased array: Crystals grouped into a cluster under a flat footprint. Timed electrical impulses sent to each crystal in specific sequences that form a wedge-shaped image. Most often used for cardiac imaging.

- Ultrasound console: Varies depending on the manufacturer. However, the clinician only needs to identify two important controls to get started.
  - Depth: Allows increase or decrease in the depth of signal penetration. Depth markers are located on the right side of the screen and demarcated in centimeters. To improve focus and resolution, adjust so that the item of interest is occupying the middle of the screen.
  - Gain: Affects overall screen brightness through the amplification of returning signals. Increasing gain increases the screen brightness but does not improve resolution.
- Additional helpful controls
  - Time Gain Compensation (TGC): Allows differential brightness control at varying depths. Allows for finer control to compensate for signal attenuation at greater depths. Increasing the TGC does not improve resolution.
  - Freeze: Allows the sonographer to freeze a screen image, usually for saving or printing.
  - Color: A bidirectional form of Doppler ultrasound which represents items moving toward the direction of the probe in one color and items moving away from the probe in another color. The color scale is usually located on the left of the image; colors at the top of the scale are moving toward the probe and colors at the bottom are moving away. This is most frequently used for evaluation of vascular structures.
  - Presets: Most machines have pre-programmed settings for acoustic power, gain, and other controls for different applications (for example, a "cardiac" preset for imaging the heart). Start with these presets and make adjustments as needed.
- Orientation: Similar to other imaging modalities, ultrasound images are oriented in consistent format to facilitate image interpretation by different clinicians.
  - Transducers will have a "probe indicator" on one side. This corresponds to a "screen indicator" visible on the left or right of the display.
  - In most imaging studies in CUS, the screen indicator is on the left side of the US image when viewed by the clinician.
  - Additionally, the probe indicator is always pointed either up to the patient's head or to the patient right side. For example, when viewing the aorta in long axis, the probe indicator is pointed toward the patient's head (*). Therefore, the more proximal portion of the aorta is viewed on the left side of the US screen (*).

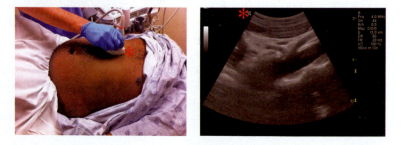

- When viewing the aorta in the short axis, the probe indicator (*) is pointed toward the patient's right. Therefore, the patient's right side is viewed on the left side of the US screen (*).

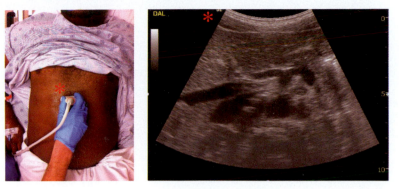

- For cardiac imaging, the orientation is often reversed. The screen indicator is on the right side of the screen. Although the optimal convention remains a source of great debate, the most important consideration is that the clinician understands the screen orientation and underlying anatomy.

PROCEDURAL CONSIDERATIONS

- Dynamic versus static approach:
  - Dynamic approach: Procedure performed under direct ultrasound visualization.
  - Static approach: Anatomy is first mapped with ultrasound and entry point marked. Procedure then performed using skin markings alone.
  - Decision on which approach used is based on clinical scenario and operator preference.
- Dual versus single operator dynamic approach options:
  - Dual operator: One clinician performs the ultrasound while the second performs the procedure under direct visualization. Easier to master for novice sonographers.
  - Single operator: One clinician performs the ultrasound and procedure concurrently.
  - This requires more skill and experience but provides finer degree of control.
- In plane versus out of plane:
  - For ultrasound guided procedures involving needle insertion, such as abscess aspiration and pericardiocentesis, in plane refers to the visualization of the entire long axis of the needle within the ultrasound beam.
  - Out of plane refers to the visualization of only a cross section of the needle passing through the ultrasound beam.

The Editors

Tarina Lee Kang, MD
Director of Emergency Ultrasound
Department of Emergency Medicine
LAC and USC Medical Center
Los Angeles, California

John Bailitz, MD
Emergency Ultrasound Division Director
Department of Emergency Medicine
Cook County Hospital
Chicago, Illinois

Contributing Authors

Gavin Budhram, MD
Chief, Emergency Ultrasound
Baystate Medical Center
Springfield, Massachusetts

Mikaela Chilstrom, MD
Division of Emergency Ultrasound
LAC+USC Medical Center
Los Angeles, California

Karen S. Cosby, MD
Emergency Ultrasound Director
Cook County Hospital
Chicago, Illinois

Robert Ehrman, MD
Emergency Ultrasound Fellow
Cook County Hospital
Chicago, Illinois

Joy English, MD
Sports Medicine and Emergency
    Ultrasound Faculty
Washington University
St. Louis, Missouri

Dasia Esener, MD
Staff Physician
Kaiser Permanente
San Diego, California

Nadim Hafez, MD
Director, Emergency Ultrasound
Rush Medical Center
Chicago, Illinois

Russ Horowitz, MD
Pediatric Emergency Ultrasound
    Director
Lurie Children's Hospital
Chicago, Illinois

John Jesus, MD
Emergency Medicine Academic
    Faculty
Christiana Hospital
Wilmington, Delaware

John Lemos
Kaiser Permanente South Sacramento
Sacramento, California

Christopher Lim, MD
Staff Physician
Department of Emergency Medicine
Cook County Hospital
Chicago, Illinois

Danielle McGee, MD
Emergency Ultrasound Faculty
Northwestern University
Chicago, Illinois

Roderick Roxas, MD
Emergency Ultrasound Director
Community Hospital of the Monterey
    Peninsula
Monterey, California

Frances Russell, MD
Emergency Ultrasound Faculty
Indiana University
Indianapolis, Indiana

Katie Tataris, MD, MPH
Emergency Medicine
University of Chicago
Chicago, Illinois

1 Trauma

John Bailitz

INDICATIONS

- Evaluate blunt or penetrating trauma to torso for intra-abdominal or intra-thoracic bleeding
- Perform serial abdominal exams for new or progressive bleeding
- Assess for pneumothorax of any etiology

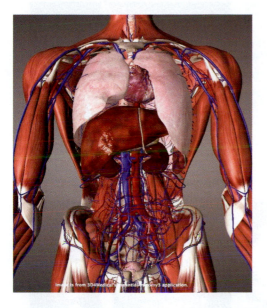

IMAGE ACQUISITION AND INTERPRETATION

EQUIPMENT

- Phased array or curvilinear 2.5–5 MHz transducer

PREPARATION

- Perform prior to Foley placement to utilize the bladder as an acoustic window.
- Place the patient supine or in slight Trendelenburg when possible to increase the amount of dependent fluid in the hepatorenal fossa (Morison's pouch).

RECOMMENDED VIEWS

Order determined by clinical context.

1. Subxiphoid
2. Right upper quadrant
3. Left upper quadrant
4. Pelvis
5. Thorax

SUBXIPHOID VIEW

TRANSDUCER PLACEMENT

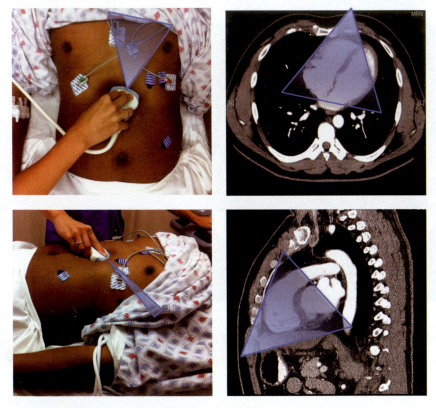

- To visualize the pericardium, place the transducer in the transverse scanning plane just to the right of the xiphoid process aiming toward the left scapula with the indicator toward the patient's right.
- With inadequate visualization, increase your depth and ask the patient to take a breath and hold in to bring the mediastinum toward the transducer.
- If view obscured by stomach gas, slide the transducer to patient's right slightly, to use more of the liver as an acoustic window.
- A minority of patients require a parasternal long view.

NORMAL ANATOMY

Top of image to bottom:

a. Left lobe of the liver
b. Anterior pericardium
c. Right ventricle
d. Septum
e. Left ventricle
f. Posterior pericardium

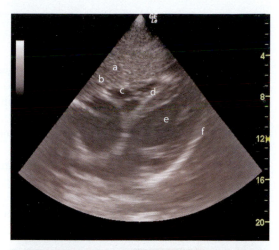

PATHOLOGY

- Acute bleeding is visualized as an anechoic fluid collection within the pericardial sac, between the visceral and parietal anterior and posterior pericardium (*).
- With increasing bleeding, fluid surrounds the heart, becoming visible in the anterior pericardium.
- With time, clotting results with mixed echogenicity.

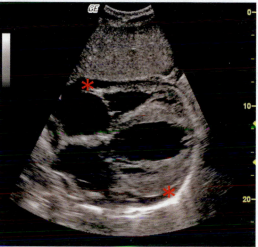

- The noncompliant pericardial sac may quickly tamponade venous return, visualized as diastolic right heart collapse (*), especially in the hypovolemic patient.
- A benign anterior pericardial fat pad will have a mixed echogenicity, not seen posteriorly or changing on repeat exam.

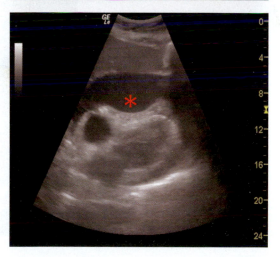

RIGHT UPPER QUADRANT VIEW

TRANSDUCER POSITION

- To visualize Morison's pouch, place the transducer in the mid-axillary line in the coronal scanning plane, in the 9th to 11th intercostal space, aiming obliquely toward the retroperitoneum with the indicator pointing toward the patient's head.
- Avoid rib shadows by slightly rotating indicator toward the bed in an oblique plane.
- To better visualize the subphrenic space and right thorax, slide the transducer up an intercostal space, or ask the patient to take a deep breath in and hold for 5 seconds. Alternatively, slide the transducer more anteriorly toward the axillary line at the 8th to 9th intercostal space, again fanning toward the retroperitoneum.

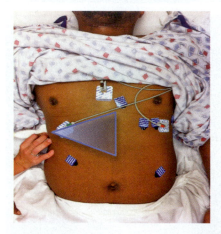
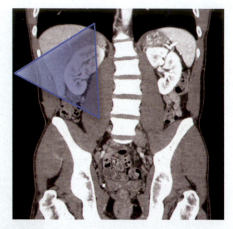

NORMAL ANATOMY

Left to right of image:

- a. Thorax
- b. Diaphragm
- c. Liver
- d. Morison's pouch
- e. Right kidney

PATHOLOGY

- Acute bleeding will fill the pelvis, then spill over the right paracolic gutter into Morison's pouch, the most dependent portion of the abdomen above the pelvis.

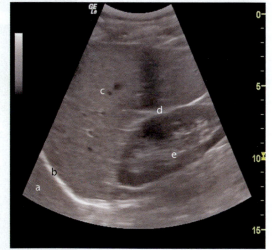

- Fluid (*) will appear as an anechoic fluid collection below the diaphragm (*).
- Anechoic fluid may represent acute bleeding, urine from a bladder rupture, or pre-existing ascites. Serial exams and other tests will clarify.

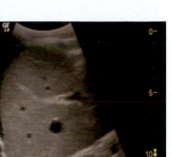

LEFT UPPER QUADRANT VIEW

TRANSDUCER POSITION

- To visualize the splenorenal space, place the transducer in the posterior axillary line in the coronal scanning plane, in the 8th to 10th intercostal space, aiming obliquely toward the retroperitoneum with the indicator pointing toward the patient's head. The probe should be more superior and posterior than in the right upper quadrant view.

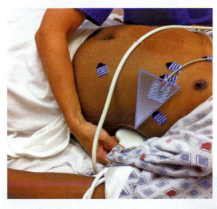
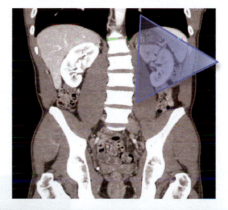

NORMAL ANATOMY

Left to right of image:

a. Diaphragm
b. Subphrenic space
c. Spleen
d. Splenorenal space
e. Left kidney

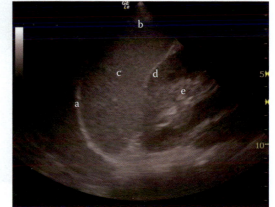

PATHOLOGY

- Acute bleeding will collect in the subphrenic space in the left upper quadrant. The higher left paracolic gutter, phrenicocolic ligament, and splenic hilum prevent blood from easily collecting in the splenorenal space (*).

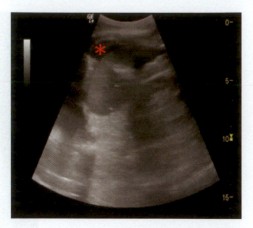

PELVIS

TRANSDUCER POSITION

- Perform the exam prior to Foley placement in order to utilize the filled bladder as an acoustic window to more posterior structures.
- To visualize the retrouterine Pouch of Douglas, or retrovesicular space in males, place the transducer just above the pubic symphysis in the midline of the abdomen in the longitudinal scanning plane.
- Rotate the transducer 90 degrees to the patient's right to visualize the structures in short axis.

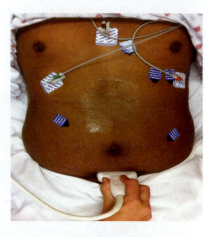

NORMAL ANATOMY

Top to bottom of image:

    a. Bladder
    b. Retrovesicular space
    c. Pouch of Douglas

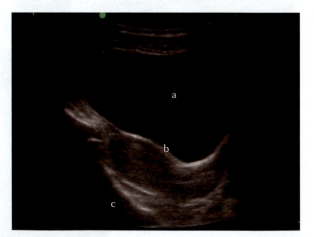

PATHOLOGY

- Blood will fill the pelvis, the most dependent portion of the peritoneal cavity, before spilling into the right upper and ultimately left upper quadrants (*).
- Be sure that blood posterior to the bladder is not obscured by high gain settings.

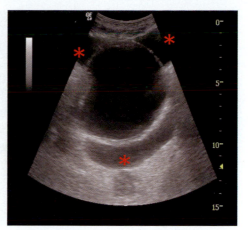

THORAX

TRANSDUCER POSITION

- To visualize normal lung sliding at the pleural line, place the transducer in the 2nd or 3rd intercostal space, at the midclavicular line, in the longitudinal scanning plane, and decrease depth.
- For equivocal cases, utilize color flow, power Doppler, or M-mode to improve visualization of horizontal pleural movement.
- Slide the transducer inferiorly and laterally 1–2 intercostal spaces and visualize the pleural line, until reaching the 6th intercostal space in the posterior axillary line.

NORMAL ANATOMY

Left to right of image:

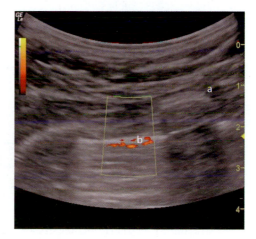

a. Rib cross-section
b. Pleural line just beneath rib

PATHOLOGY

- Normal lung sliding rules out a pneumothorax.
- Loss of normal lung sliding in the trauma patient suggests a pneumothorax, but may also occur with pleural blebs in patients with emphysema, hypoventilation due to right main stem intubation, or patients with prior pleural scarring.

- Visualization of the lung point, where the parietal and visceral pleura are still intermittently apposed, is diagnostic of pneumothorax.
- M-mode imaging will reveal a seashore sign (waves/barcode crashing on the grainy beach of lung artifact—lower left) of the normal lung, and only a barcode over the pneumothorax (lower right *).

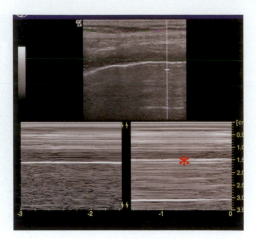

INTEGRATION OF FINDINGS

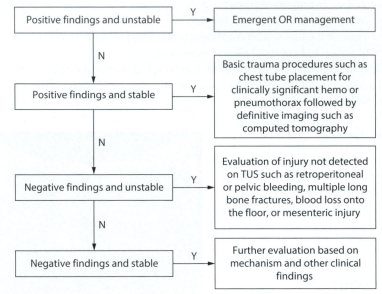

Positive findings and unstable	**Y** → Emergent OR management
N ↓	
Positive findings and stable	**Y** → Basic trauma procedures such as chest tube placement for clinically significant hemo or pneumothorax followed by definitive imaging such as computed tomography
N ↓	
Negative findings and unstable	**Y** → Evaluation of injury not detected on TUS such as retroperitoneal or pelvic bleeding, multiple long bone fractures, blood loss onto the floor, or mesenteric injury
N ↓	
Negative findings and stable	**Y** → Further evaluation based on mechanism and other clinical findings

SPECIAL CONSIDERATIONS

- Trauma for pediatric patients has yielded less and sometimes conflicting data. Recent studies demonstrate a high specificity but low sensitivity. When positive, the exam may be helpful. When negative, additional studies are still needed. Additionally, pediatric solid organ injury is more often managed non-operatively compared to adults. However, this rapid diagnostic tool still provides valuable information in the often easy-to-scan unstable pediatric multisystem trauma patient.

2 Echo and IVC

Roderick Roxas and John Jesus

INDICATIONS

Evaluate for suspected pericardial effusion, tamponade, right heart strain, impaired ejection fraction, hypovolemia, or hypervolemia.

IMAGE ACQUISITION AND INTERPRETATION

EQUIPMENT

- Small footprint phased array 2.5–5 MHz transducer

PREPARATION

- To optimize image acquisition, lie patient flat.
- If patient unable to lie flat, then scan patient with the head of the bed elevated 15–30 degrees in left lateral decubitus position. (Although the chapter images show the screen indicator on both the left and right side, cardiology conventions using the cardiology preset will be utilized.)

RECOMMENDED VIEWS

- Subxiphoid (SX)
- Parasternal Long Axis (PLAX)
- Parasternal Short Axis (PSAX)
- Apical 4 Chamber (A4C)

SUBXIPHOID

TRANSDUCER PLACEMENT

- To obtain a subxiphoid view of the heart, first place the transducer in the coronal plane under the xiphoid process with the probe marker pointing toward the patient's left side. Angle the ultrasound beam "under" the sternum aiming at the left scapula until the following image is obtained.

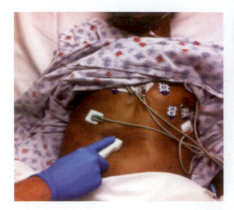
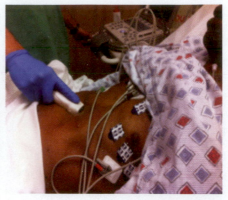

NORMAL ANATOMY

Top of image to bottom:

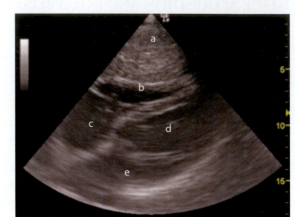

a. Left lobe of the liver
b. Right ventricle
c. Right atrium
d. Left ventricle
e. Left atrium

PATHOLOGY

- Utilize the subcostal view to assess for pericardial effusion and cardiac tamponade.
- In the recumbent patient, pericardial effusions will be visualized as anechoic fluid collections deep to the posterior wall of the left ventricle. Larger effusions will wrap around into the anterior pericardial space (*).

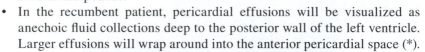

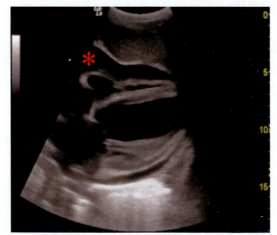

- An anterior pericardial fat pad can mimic the appearance of a pericardial effusion. Pericardial fat pads at times have a mixed, "dirty" echogenicity and move with cardiac activity, while pericardial effusions are usually anechoic and do not move with cardiac activity.
- Cardiac tamponade is demonstrated when the right ventricle collapses (*) during diastole in the presence of a pericardial effusion.

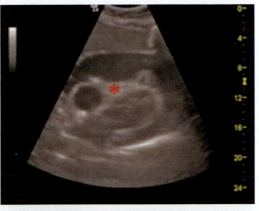

PARASTERNAL LONG AXIS

TRANSDUCER PLACEMENT

- To obtain a parasternal long view of the heart, place the probe immediately adjacent to the left side of the sternum in the 4th intercostal space with the probe marker pointing toward the patient's right shoulder.
- Once the heart is seen, adjust the probe position in the same intercostal space to improve the view.

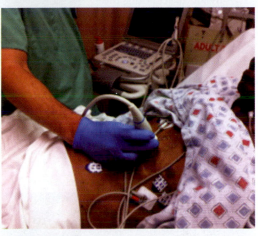

NORMAL ANATOMY

Top of image to bottom, and left to right:

a. Lung
b. Right ventricle
c. Left ventricular outflow tract and aortic root
d. Left ventricle, mitral valve, and left atrium
e. Posterior pericardium
f. Descending aorta

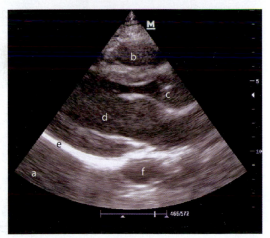

PATHOLOGY

- Utilize the PLAX to qualitatively assess the ejection fraction. In a normal heart, the septal and posterior walls of the left ventricle will literally squeeze together. Additionally, the anterior leaflet of the mitral valve will appear to touch the septum.
- A normal aortic root is less than 3.5 cm. A flap may be seen arising from the root in type A dissections. A flap may also be seen in the short axis view of the aorta in the far field of the PLAX image.
- In the supine patient, pericardial effusions can be visualized as anechoic fluid collections deep to the posterior wall of the left ventricle.
- Pleural effusions (*) can mimic the appearance of a pericardial effusion. Pericardial effusions cross anterior to the descending thoracic aorta, while pleural effusions do not.

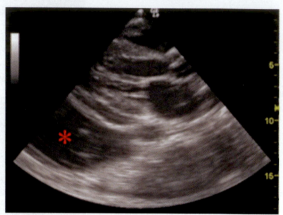

PARASTERNAL SHORT AXIS

TRANSDUCER PLACEMENT

- To obtain a parasternal short view of the heart, first obtain the PLAX view as above. Center the left ventricle in the middle of the screen. From there, rotate the transducer 90 degrees clockwise until the probe marker is roughly pointing toward the patient's left shoulder and the left ventricle is circular in shape.

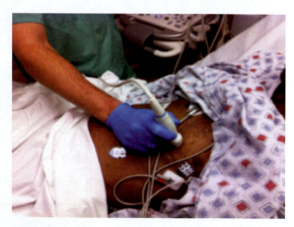

- Angle the probe either medially or laterally until the papillary muscles are visualized.

NORMAL ANATOMY

Top of image to bottom:

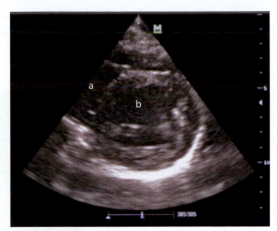

a. Right ventricle
b. Left ventricle and papillary muscles

PATHOLOGY

- Utilize the PSAX to qualitatively assess the ejection fraction. This must be done at the level of the papillary muscles to be accurate.
- With each contraction, the myocardium should concentrically change thickness resulting in an obvious reduction in ventricular cavity size.
- The PSAX is superior to the PLAX when assessing the ejection fraction. This eliminates the chance of an oblique image through the left ventricle overestimating the ejection fraction.
- Paradoxical movement of the inter-ventricular septum into the left ventricle during systole, creating a D shape (*), suggests right ventricular strain.

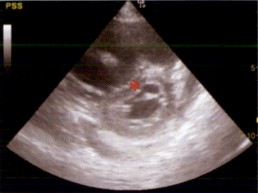

APICAL 4 CHAMBER

TRANSDUCER PLACEMENT

- To obtain an A4C view of the heart, place the transducer at the point of maximal impulse within the 5th to 6th intercostal space in the transverse plane with the probe marker pointing toward the patient's left side or the bed. Angle the ultrasound beam cephalad until all 4 chambers of the

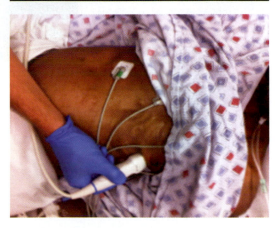

heart are visualized in a single image. Slide laterally if necessary until the septum travels down the middle of the screen.
- To optimize the A4C view, place the patient in left lateral decubitus if clinically feasible.

Normal Anatomy

Top of image to bottom, left side to right side:

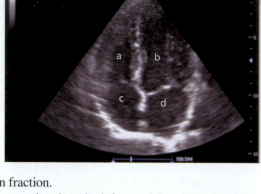

a. Right ventricle
b. Left ventricle
c. Right atrium
d. Left atrium

Pathology

- Utilize the A4C view to qualitatively assess the ejection fraction.
- A right ventricle equal to or larger size than the left ventricle suggests right ventricular strain. The A4C view is the optimal view to compare right to left heart size. In 10–15% of cases, a massive PE (*) may be seen in the right heart.
- Chronic strain on the right ventricle often seen with chronic pulmonary hypertension results in right ventricular hypertrophy, suggested by a wall thickness greater than 0.5 cm.

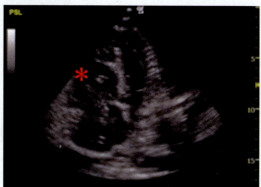

- McConnell sign, akinesis of the mid-portion of the right ventricular free wall, yet normal contraction of the right ventricular apex suggests acute pulmonary embolism.

IVC ASSESSMENT

Equipment

- Curvilinear or phased array probe

PREPARATION

- Place the patient in the supine position if possible.

RECOMMENDED VIEWS

- Transverse view or longitudinal view of the IVC

TRANSVERSE VIEW

TRANSDUCER PLACEMENT

- Place the probe in the transverse position just caudal to the xiphoid process.

NORMAL ANATOMY

- The IVC is on the anatomical right; the aorta is on the anatomical left; both lie anterior to the vertebral body.
- The IVC will compress in response to direct pressure, while the aorta will not.

LONGITUDINAL VIEW

TRANSDUCER PLACEMENT

- Center the IVC on the ultrasound screen. With the probe maintaining contact with the patient's abdomen, turn the probe to the sagittal position with the indicator pointed cephalad.

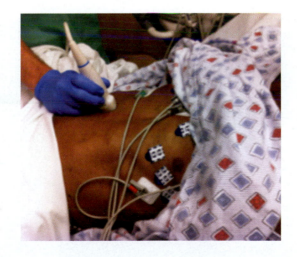

NORMAL ANATOMY

Top of image to bottom:

 a. Liver
 b. IVC

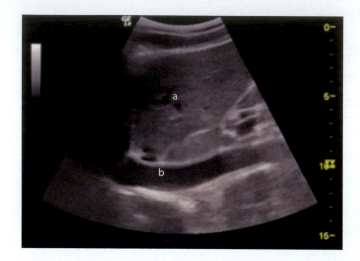

PATHOLOGY

- A small IVC (*) is typically less than 1.5 cm.
- Complete respiratory collapse of the IVC suggests a central venous pressure (CVP) of <8 and the need for aggressive resuscitation in the setting of hypovolemic or distributive shock.

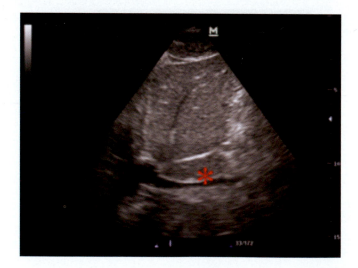

- A large IVC (*), typically greater than 2.5 cm, with minimal respiratory variation suggests a diagnosis of congestive heart failure (CHF). Additional fluid administration is unlikely to be helpful and may lead to fluid overload.

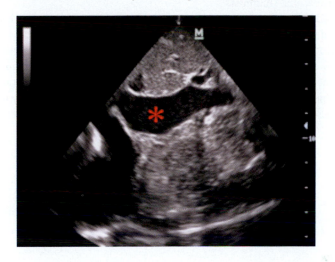

INTEGRATION OF FINDINGS

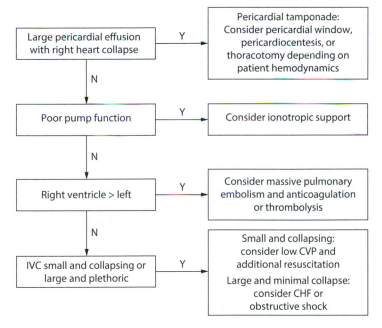

Large pericardial effusion with right heart collapse	Y →	Pericardial tamponade: Consider pericardial window, pericardiocentesis, or thoracotomy depending on patient hemodynamics
↓ N		
Poor pump function	Y →	Consider ionotropic support
↓ N		
Right ventricle > left	Y →	Consider massive pulmonary embolism and anticoagulation or thrombolysis
↓ N		
IVC small and collapsing or large and plethoric	Y →	Small and collapsing: consider low CVP and additional resuscitation Large and minimal collapse: consider CHF or obstructive shock

SPECIAL CONSIDERATIONS

- In a patient with undifferentiated shock, limited bedside echo helps narrow the differential diagnosis.
- With adequate training, emergency physicians' classification of low versus normal ejection fraction correlates well with cardiologists'.
- The limitations of using CVP for the evaluation of volume status also exist for US evaluation of the IVC and CI. Pathology that results in an increase in right heart pressures such as acute obstructive shock states (pulmonary embolus, tamponade, tension pneumothorax), chronic pulmonary hypertension, and others may reduce the reliability and utility of CVP.

3 Lung

Roderick Roxas

INDICATIONS

- Evaluate undifferentiated dyspnea suggestive of either cardiac or lung disease

IMAGE ACQUISITION AND INTERPRETATION

EQUIPMENT

- Phased array or curvilinear 2.5–5 MHz transducer

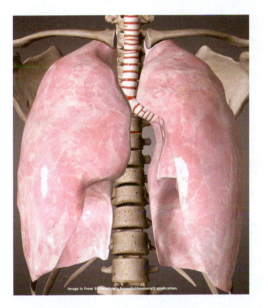

Image is from 3D4Medical's EssentialAnatomy5 application.

PREPARATION

- For pleural scanning, set depth to 6–8 cm. For pneumothorax, please see Chapter 1, Trauma.
- For lung scanning, set the depth to 18 cm.
- Turn off all image post-processing on your US system such as harmonics and cross-beam, which may remove the artifacts necessary to identify normal and abnormal lung.

RECOMMENDED VIEWS

- Divide each hemithorax into four quadrants. First, visualize a square bordered by the sternum and the posterior axillary line, clavicle and costal margin. Then section into superior and inferior halves at the nipple line, followed by anterior and posterior quadrants at the anterior axillary line.

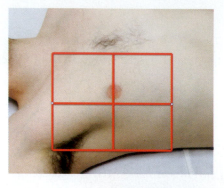

TRANSDUCER PLACEMENT

- Place the transducer in the sagittal scanning plane in each quadrant.
- There is no mandate on the order in which views are performed.

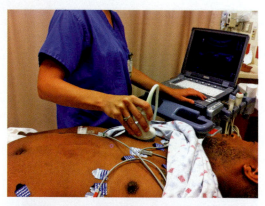

NORMAL ANATOMY

a. The hyperechoic pleural line may be connecting the posterior borders of adjacent ribs.

b. A-lines (*) are horizontal, bright, hyperechoic reflections of the pleural line that repeat at equal intervals.

c. B-lines are vertical, bright, hyperechoic, laser-like artifacts that radiate from the pleural line to the end of the image without diminishing. B-lines erase A-lines as they traverse the image.

d. One or two B-lines in a scanning quadrant can be normal, particularly in the lung bases.

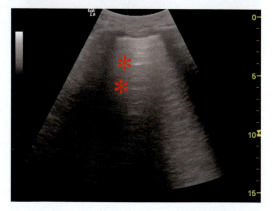

PATHOLOGY

- An increase in the number of B-lines (*) results from interlobular septal thickening. This may result from several different disease processes including congestive heart failure (most common in the ED), interstitial lung disease, and ARDS.
- Early interstitial edema can be detected when three or more B-lines are visualized in two or more scanning quadrants, bilaterally.

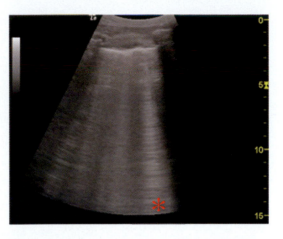

- As edema increases, adjacent B-lines coalesce to form bright bands.

INTEGRATION OF FINDINGS

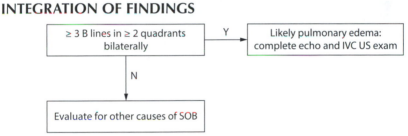

SPECIAL CONSIDERATIONS

- Thoracic ultrasound rapidly assesses for pulmonary edema in the correct clinical scenario.

4 Abdominal Aorta

Roderick Roxas

INDICATIONS

- Assess back, flank, chest, or abdominal pain suggestive of abdominal aortic aneurysm or dissection
- Assess for suspected urinary retention

IMAGE ACQUISITION AND INTERPRETATION

EQUIPMENT

- Curvilinear 2.5–5 MHz probe. If not available, then phased array probe

PREPARATION

- Place patient in the supine position.
- Place gel in the midline of the abdomen from the xiphoid process to the umbilicus.

RECOMMENDED VIEWS

- Short axis of the proximal aorta
- Short axis of the distal abdominal aorta
- Long axis of the proximal abdominal aorta
- Long axis of the distal abdominal aorta

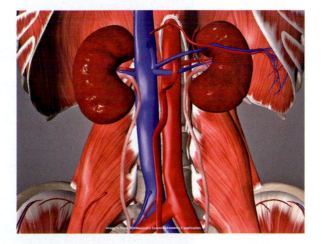

SHORT AXIS OF THE PROXIMAL ABDOMINAL AORTA

TRANSDUCER PLACEMENT

- To evaluate the proximal abdominal aorta in its short axis, place the transducer in the transverse plane over the epigastrium with the probe marker pointing toward the patient's right side.

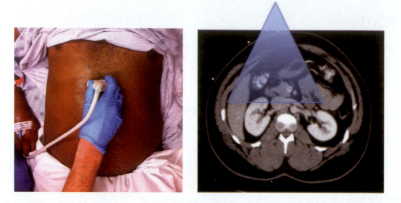

- Slide the probe caudad until you achieve either of the two images below, confirming placement over the proximal portion of the abdominal aorta.

NORMAL ANATOMY

Top of image to bottom, left to right:

At celiac artery
   a. Left lobe of liver
   b. Celiac artery
   c. IVC (teardrop)
   d. Aorta (circular)
   e. Vertebral body with vertebral shadowing

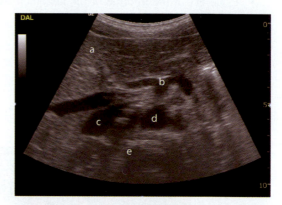

At superior mesenteric artery
   a. Portosplenic vein
   b. Superior mesenteric artery (mantle clock)
   c. Aorta

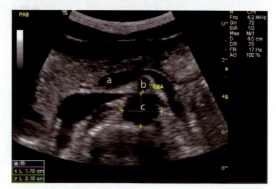

SHORT AXIS OF THE DISTAL ABDOMINAL AORTA

Transducer Placement

- First obtain the short axis view of the proximal abdominal aorta as above.
- Then continue to visualize the aorta in its short axis as you lift and press the transducer distally in 1-centimeter increments to displace bowel gas until reaching the bifurcation of the common iliac arteries.
- Obtain images of the abdominal aorta just proximal to the bifurcation.

Normal Anatomy

- Aorta
- Inferior vena cava

LONG AXIS OF THE PROXIMAL ABDOMINAL AORTA

Transducer Placement

- From the proximal short axis view, rotate the transducer 90 degrees clockwise until the probe marker is pointing toward the patient's head.
- The abdominal aorta is now visualized as a long tubular structure with the following vessels branching off.

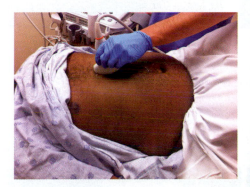
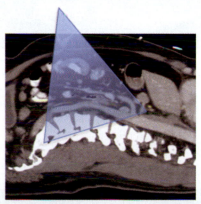

Normal Anatomy

Top of image to bottom, left to right:

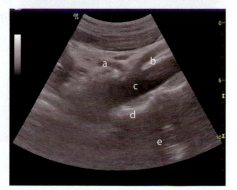

- a. Celiac trunk
- b. Superior mesenteric artery
- c. Aorta
- d. Vertebral body (bright scalloped lines posterior to the aorta)

LONG AXIS OF THE DISTAL ABDOMINAL AORTA

Transducer Placement

- From the proximal long axis view, lift and press the transducer as above to visualize the entire course of the aorta below the bifurcation and the proximal portion of both iliac arteries.

Pathology

- The abdominal aorta is normally <3 cm in diameter measured from outer wall to inner wall. Be careful to measure only the true lumen of a large abdominal aortic aneurysm (AAA) (*).
- The risk of rupture increases as the size of the aneurysm increases especially when greater than 5 cm.

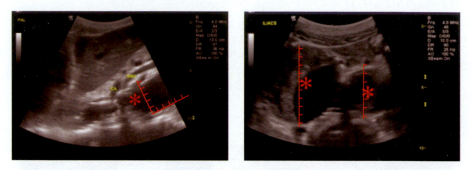

- AAA can rupture either into the peritoneal cavity (immediate exsanguination) or the retroperitoneum (may occur more slowly). Ultrasound is not sensitive for detecting retroperitoneal rupture.
- When an AAA is detected in a hypotensive patient, assume rupture until proven otherwise.
- An undulating flap inside the aortic lumen may be better seen on the long axis view of the aorta (*).

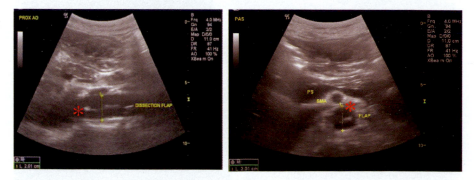

- Additionally, check the parasternal long axis view to visualize the aortic root and the descending thoracic aorta for aneurysm and dissection.

INTEGRATION OF FINDINGS

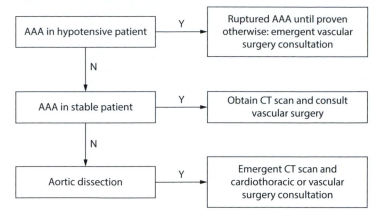

SPECIAL CONSIDERATIONS

- In a patient with undifferentiated shock, bedside ultrasound evaluation of the abdominal aorta helps narrow the differential diagnosis.
- Bedside ultrasound is 100% sensitive for detecting an abdominal aortic aneurysm if the entire length of the abdominal aorta is visualized.
- Bowel gas may obscure portions of the abdominal aorta. Continuously lift and press with firm pressure over these areas to help move the bowel gas.
- If that is not successful, consider scanning the aorta from just off center or via a coronal view from the right upper quadrant.
- Bedside ultrasound is specific but not sensitive for aortic dissection.

5 Renal and Bladder

Christopher Lim

INDICATIONS

- Evaluate pain suggestive of renal colic
- Measure post-void residual bladder volume

IMAGE ACQUISITION AND INTERPRETATION

EQUIPMENT

- A low frequency 3–6 MHz curvilinear or phased array transducer

PREPARATION

- Place patient in supine position.
- Consider the lateral decubitus position when imaging the kidneys if needed.
- Ensure patient is well hydrated prior to evaluation for hydronephrosis.
- Prepare to measure post-void residual immediately after voiding attempt.

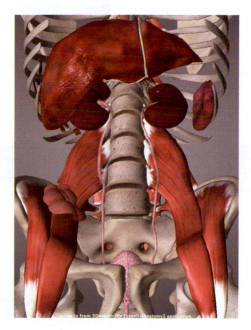

RECOMMENDED VIEWS

1. Both kidneys in the transverse and horizontal planes
2. The bladder in the transverse and horizontal planes

KIDNEY LONG AND SHORT VIEWS

TRANSDUCER PLACEMENT

- Place the transducer in the mid-axillary line, in the 10th–12th intercostal space or below, with the indicator on the probe toward the patient's head in the coronal plane.

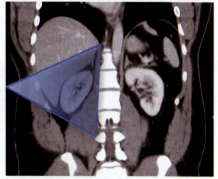

- Turn the probe at a slightly oblique angle to fit the probe head within the plane of the intercostal space to visualize the kidney in the kidney's long axis.
- Improve visualization of the kidney by asking the patient to take a deep breath and hold for 5 to 10 seconds to open the intercostal space and displace kidney inferiorly.

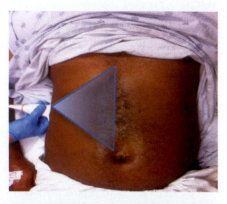

- Turn the probe 90 degrees counter-clockwise to visualize the kidney in the short axis.
- Make broad sweeps in the superior/inferior and anterior/posterior planes to the entire organ.

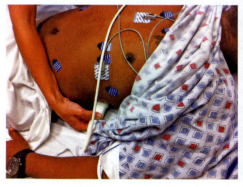

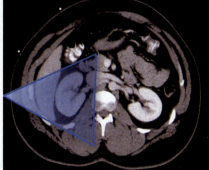

RIGHT KIDNEY

- Use the liver as an acoustic window.
- The right kidney is located more anteriorly than the left, and can usually be visualized when the probe is placed in the mid-axillary line.

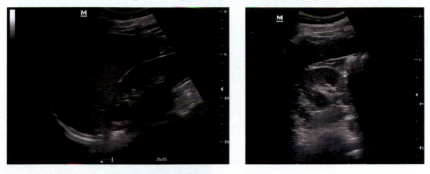

LEFT KIDNEY

- Use the spleen as an acoustic window.
- The left kidney is located more posterior and cephalad due to the smaller size of the spleen. As per the trauma LUQ view, begin with your knuckles on the bed when scanning the left kidney.

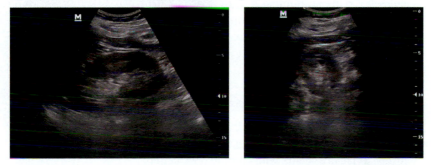

NORMAL ANATOMY

- The right kidney is bound by the liver anteriorly and cephalad, and the psoas muscle posteriorly.
- The left kidney is bound by the spleen anteriorly and cephalad, and the stomach/bowel inferiorly and anteriorly.
- Kidneys appear as bean-shaped structures in the long axis and C-shaped structures in the short axis.
- The central portion of the kidney formed by the calyces and renal pelvis is normally hyperechoic.
- The surrounding renal parenchyma is composed of the medulla and cortex and normally appears hypoechoic.
- The kidney is surrounded by a dense hyperechoic fibrous capsule known as Gerota's fascia.

- Benign renal cysts appear as thin-walled, round structures at the periphery of the renal cortex without internal echoes.
- Triangular medullary pyramids can be distinguished from hydronephrosis by the presence of renal parenchyma between adjacent pyramids and the absence of connection with the renal pelvis.

PATHOLOGY

- Anechoic areas within the renal pelvis and calyces suggests hydronephrosis.
- Hydronephrosis can be graded as mild, moderate, or severe.
- Mild (*)—Subtle prominence of calyces often only detected after comparison views. Use color flow to ensure that the renal artery and vein are not being mistaken for hydronephrosis.

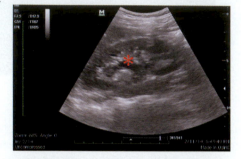

- Moderate (*)—Dilation of calyces and pelvis without thinning of the renal cortex. Obvious even before comparison.

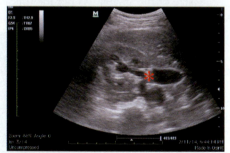

- Severe (*)—Markedly distended calyces and pelvis with thinning of renal cortex. Typically occurs with chronic obstruction.

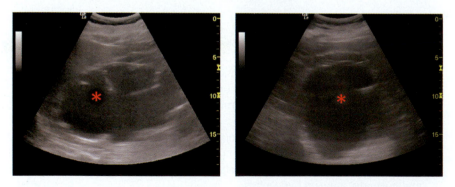

- Renal stones appear as dense hyperechoic structures with posterior shadowing. Twinkle artifact may be seen posterior to the stone with color flow imaging.

BLADDER VIEWS

- Place transducer just above pubic symphysis, with the indicator on the probe toward the patient's right.
- Angle the probe face toward the patient's feet to visualize the pelvis.
- Rotate the transducer 90 degrees to obtain the longitudinal view.

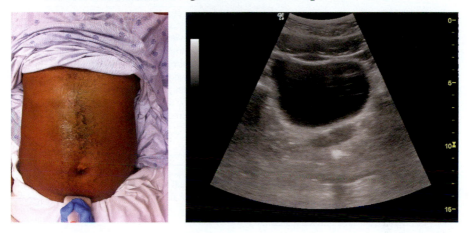

NORMAL ANATOMY

- The bladder appears as an anechoic cavity in the pelvis.
- The prostate is visualized posterior and caudal to the bladder. The uterus is visualized posterior and cephalad to the bladder.
- If not automatically measured by the machine, estimate bladder volume with the following formula with a correction factor for the ellipsoid shape of the bladder:

$$\text{Volume bladder} = 0.75 \times \text{width} \times \text{length} \times \text{height in mm}$$

PATHOLOGY

- Bladder outlet obstruction: will appear as a persistently full bladder (>100–150 mL) after attempted urinary voiding.

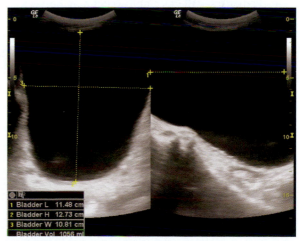

INTEGRATION OF FINDINGS

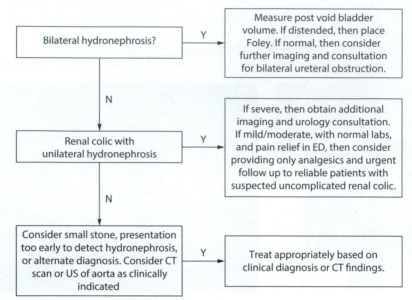

SPECIAL CONSIDERATIONS

- A large AAA may compress the ureter with resultant hydronephrosis. The most common misdiagnosis for an AAA is "renal colic." Always consider AAA as a diagnosis and visualize the aorta in any patient over 45 or with risk factors for AAA who presents with first-time flank, abdominal, or back pain.
- Pregnancy—The gravid fetus exerts pressure on ureters, and hydronephrosis may be a normal finding often more pronounced on the right due to the slightly right-sided position of the typical gravid uterus.
- Pediatrics—Bladder ultrasound may be very useful in deciding when and how to preform bladder catheterization.
- Prostatitis—Determination of ultrasound post-void residual prevents further prostate irritation and inflammation from an unnecessary straight cath.
- For any "first-time renal colic" patient older than 45, always be sure to ultrasound the aorta as well to rule out an AAA.

6 Biliary

Katie Tataris and John Bailitz

INDICATIONS

- Evaulate source of right upper quadrant, flank, epigastric pain, or sepsis without a source in a patient with altered mental status
- Assess a patient with jaundice

IMAGE ACQUISITION AND INTERPRETATION

EQUIPMENT

- Curvilinear or phased array 3.0–6.0 MHz transducer

PREPARATION

- Place patient in left lateral decubitus position.
- Instruct patient to take a deep breath and hold for 5 to 10 seconds to bring the gallbladder down below the rib margin.

RECOMMENDED VIEWS

1. Gallbladder long axis
2. Gallbladder short axis
3. Bile ducts

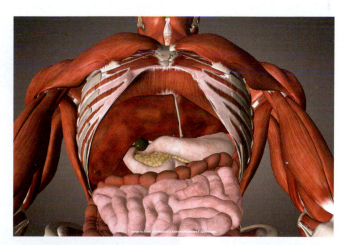

GALLBLADDER LONG AXIS

TRANSDUCER PLACEMENT

- Place the transducer in the longitudinal plane under the right costal margin at the midclavicular line with the indicator pointing toward the patient's head.

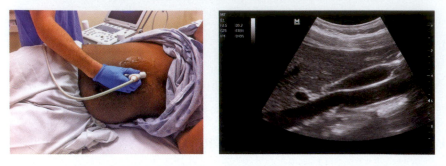

- Rock the transducer cephalad to caudad to improve visualization of the gallbladder.
- Slide the transducer medial and lateral so that the entire organ is visualized, to avoid missing stones in the more dependent portions of the gallbladder fundus.
- Use an intercostal or axillary approach if the gallbladder is not well visualized anteriorly.

NORMAL ANATOMY

Top of image to bottom, left to right:

a. The gallbladder is an anechoic, pear-shaped, cystic structure surrounded by the liver. The exact location of the gallbladder varies depending on the patient's habitus and body position.

b. The main lobar fissure (MLF) is a hyperechoic line that appears to connect the portal triad to the gallbladder.

c. Detection of the MLF and the portal triad will help distinguish a gallbladder without stones from nearby stomach, duodenum, and vasculature.

d. The portal triad consists of the portal vein (PV), common bile duct (CBD), and hepatic artery (HA). The portal triad is often called the *Mickey Mouse sign* due to appearance of the PV face, and the two ears formed by the CBD and HA (*).

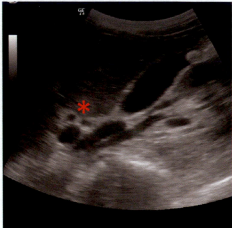

GALLBLADDER SHORT AXIS

TRANSDUCER PLACEMENT

- Turn the indicator 90 degrees counterclockwise to the patient's right.
- Slide the transducer caudad to visualize the entire gallbladder fundus. Then slide the transducer cephalad to visualize the gallbladder neck.

NORMAL ANATOMY

Top of image to bottom:

a. Measure the anterior wall of the gallbladder. Wall thickness of >3 mm suggests inflammation.
b. Wall thickening (*) may also be seen in patients who are post-prandial, or with chronic medical conditions such as CHF, renal failure, hepatitis, and cirrhosis.

PATHOLOGY

- Gallstones appear as hyperechoic, dependent foci within the lumen that cast "clean" anechoic shadows posteriorly (*).
- In contrast, polyps or masses are hyperechoic foci without shadows or movement with patient position change.
- Sludge, a precursor of stones, appears as a hypoechoic, dependent fluid that layers within the gallbladder. Sludge is often seen in patients with chronic disease.

- Acute cholecystitis: Gallstones, gallbladder wall thickening, and a sonographic Murphy sign.

- Patchy pericholecystic fluid surrounding a thickened gallbladder wall is highly specific for acute cholecystitis (*).

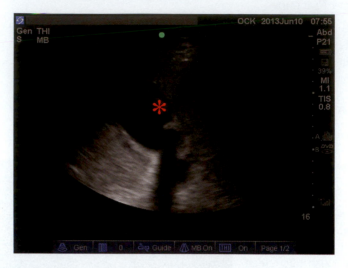

- Chronic cholecystitis: Gallstones or sludge with wall thickening, but without pericholecystic fluid or a sonographic Murphy sign.
- Acalculous cholecystitis: Gallbladder wall thickening, a sonographic Murphy sign, and pericholecystic fluid in the absence of gallstones (*).

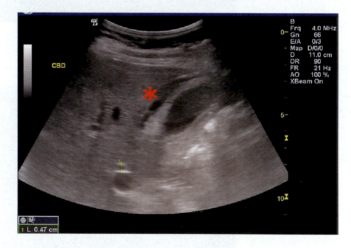

BILE DUCTS

Transducer Placement

- From the long axis of the gallbladder: The CBD is the left ear of the Mickey Mouse sign.

- From the short axis of the gallbladder: Slide the transducer cephalad to visualize the left and right portal veins with the bile duct (*).

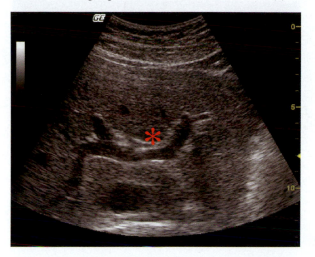

- Follow the main PV toward the umbilicus to visualize the sandwich sign formed by the CBD running anterior to the PV, which is anterior to the interior vena cava (IVC).

NORMAL ANATOMY

Top of image to bottom:

a. Measure the bile duct from inner wall to inner wall. Normal bile duct diameter is less than 6 mm, or decades in life divided by 10. Post-cholecystectomy patients may normally have a CBD up to 1 cm.

b. Within the liver, the PV has thick, hyperechoic walls while the hepatic veins have thin, invisible walls (*) and drain into the IVC.

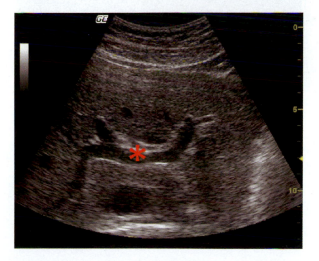

c. Use color flow to distinguish vascular from biliary structures (*).

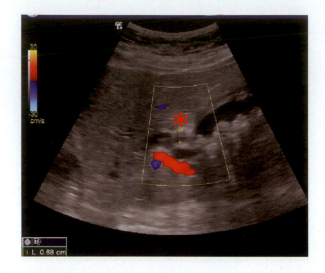

PATHOLOGY

- Bile duct enlargement is suggested by a bile duct >6 mm, and is often recognized first as:
  - Enlarged Mickey Mouse ear.
  - Double-barrel shotgun sign: A dilated bile duct (*) equal in size to the right or left PV.

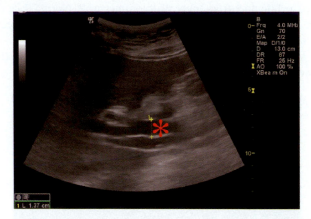

  - Antler sign: Dilated intrahepatic ducts overlying both the right and left portal veins.
- Choledocholithiasis: Stones visualized within a dilated bile duct.
- Cholangitis: Bile duct appears thickened and irregular.

INTEGRATION OF FINDINGS

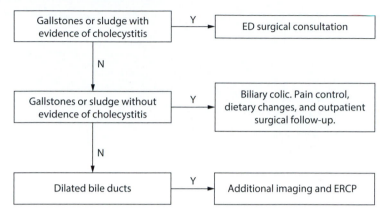

SPECIAL CONSIDERATIONS

- Pediatric cholelithiasis is rare except in patients with sickle cell disease, hemolytic anemia, or obesity.
- Geriatric and immunocompromised patients do not often present with classic signs and symptoms of biliary disease despite impressive sonographic findings.
- Always evaluate the gallbladder in septic patients without a clear source.

7 First Trimester Pregnancy

Robert Ehrman and John Bailitz

INDICATIONS

- Evaluate abdominal pain and first trimester vaginal bleeding in a patient
- Assess a female patient of childbearing age in undifferentiated shock

IMAGE ACQUISITION AND INTERPRETATION

EQUIPMENT

- Curvilinear 3–5 MHz transducer for transabdominal (TA) scanning
- Endocavitary 4–8 MHz transducer for transvaginal (TV) scanning

PREPARATION

- Transabdominal (TA) scanning:
  - Place patient in supine position.
  - Ensure that that the patient has a full bladder.
- Transvaginal (TV) scanning:
  - Place patient on pelvic exam bed.
  - Empty bladder to facilitate image acquisition.
- Cover probe with sterile condom.

RECOMMENDED VIEWS (FOR BOTH TA AND TV SCANS)

1. Uterus in long axis
2. Uterus in short axis
3. Dedicated view of pregnancy-related structures:
   a. Yolk sac/fetal pole/fetus
   b. Fetal heart rate (FHR)
   c. Gestational age estimation
   d. Adnexa (better seen on TV exams)

TRANSABDOMINAL LONGITUDINAL

TRANSDUCER PLACEMENT

- Place the probe just superior to the pubic symphysis with the indicator to the patient's head.
- Slide the probe in a left-right direction to obtain views of the entire uterus.
- Note that a full bladder is preferred for optimal image acquisition.

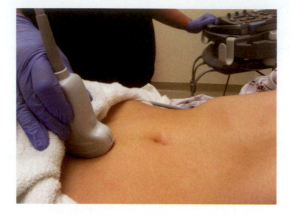

NORMAL ANATOMY

Top of image to bottom, left to right:

a. Bladder
b. Anterior uterine wall
c. Endometrial stripe/pregnancy-related structures
d. Posterior uterine wall
e. Recto-uterine pouch (Pouch of Douglas)

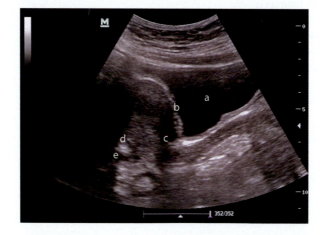

TRANSABDOMINAL TRANSVERSE

TRANSDUCER PLACEMENT

- Place the probe just superior to the pubic symphysis with the indicator to the patient's right.
- Slide the probe in a cranio-caudal direction to obtain views of the entire uterus.
- Scan in two planes to definitively locate structures in and around the uterus.

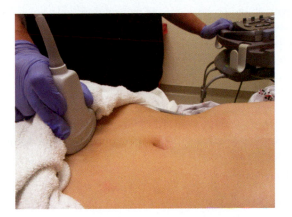

NORMAL ANATOMY

Top of image to bottom:

    a. Bladder
    b. Anterior uterine wall
    c. Endometrial stripe/pregnancy-related structures
    d. Posterior uterine wall
    e. Pouch of Douglas

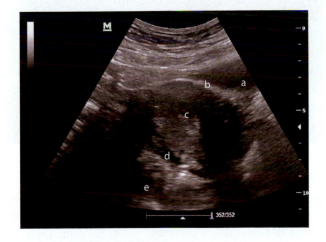

TRANSVAGINAL

- Useful adjunct in early pregnancy (5–7 weeks), as structures can be seen approximately 1 week earlier on TV US than TA.
- Considered modality of choice for basic adnexal visualization.

TRANSVAGINAL LONGITUDINAL

- Position patient and probe as for the transabdominal scan.
- View all structures in two imaging planes.
- Insert the probe with the indicator toward the ceiling.
- Fan the probe from left to right to visualize the entire uterus.
- View the cervix: Retract the probe 1–2 cm and angle the tip downward (toward patient's back).
- View the ovaries/adnexa: From the cervical view slide the probe along the lateral border of the uterus toward the left or right fornix; the ovary should come into view as you reach the deepest portions of the fornix.

NORMAL ANATOMY

Top of image to bottom, left to right:

- a. Bladder
- b. Endometrial stripe
- c. Posterior uterine wall

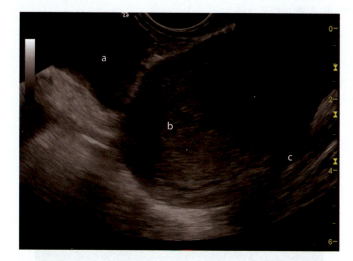

TRANSVAGINAL TRANSVERSE

- Turn the probe counterclockwise so the indicator points to the patient's right.
- Fan the probe from patient's back toward the abdominal wall to view the entire uterus and other pelvic contents.

- The fallopian tubes can be traced from the uterine cornua to aid in identification of the ovaries.
- Ovaries should be viewed in two planes to distinguish from other pelvic structures.

NORMAL ANATOMY

Top of image to bottom:

a. Anterior uterine wall (patient's feet)
b. Endometrial stripe
c. Posterior uterine wall (patient's head)

Hyperchoic area (*) = An IUD in this patient

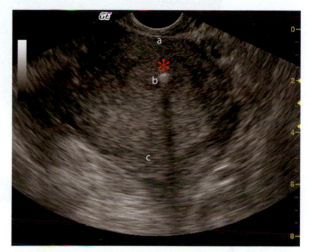

DEDICATED VIEW OF PREGNANCY-RELATED STRUCTURES

May be obtained in either plane. Structures by gestational age:

- Gestational sac (*): Earliest visible sign of pregnancy but cannot definitively diagnose intrauterine pregnancy (IUP) since a similar appearing pseudo-sac may be seen in early pregnancy. Visible at approximately 5.5 weeks TA. Fetal pole should be visible by 25 mm.

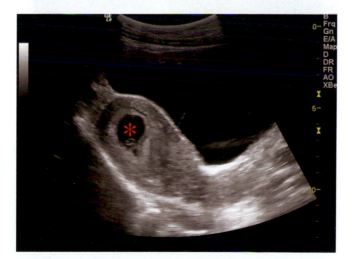

- Yolk sac (*): First definitive sign of an IUP, appears as a small ring seen within the larger gestational sac.
  - Seen at approximately 6 weeks on TA imaging.

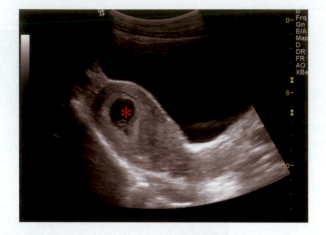

- Fetal pole (*): Echogenic structure within the gestational sac alongside the yolk sac.
  - Seen at approximately 7 weeks on TA imaging.
  - Cardiac motion may be seen within the fetal pole at this time as well.

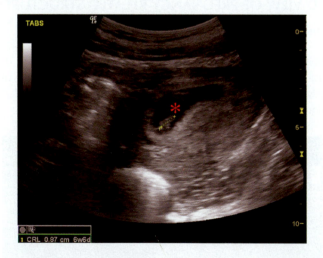

- Fetal parts: Limb buds and more developed structures can be seen from week 8 onward on TA imaging.

FETAL HEART RATE

- Place the M-mode cursor over the fetal heart.
- Cardiac motion can be seen as repeating cycles of "peaks" and "valleys."
- One cycle is measured from one peak to the next.
  - FHR can be calculated by measuring the number of cycles per second.
  - Many US machines have software that will calculate this based on the length of one or two cycles.

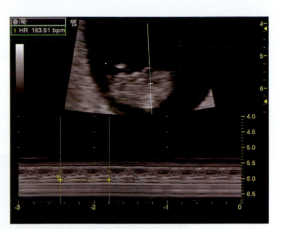

- Presence of FHR is the gold standard for diagnosing live IUP. Visible at approximately 7 weeks on TA imaging.

GESTATIONAL AGE

- Crown–rump length (CRL): Once embryo is visible, measure maximal embryo length, excluding legs and yolk sac.
- Useful in first trimester only.
- Biparietal diameter (BPD): Measure skull from outer-table to inner-table at level of ventricles.
  - Used in second trimester
  - Less accurate than CRL

ADNEXAL IMAGING

- TV images are superior to those obtained via TA route.
- Fallopian tubes arise from superiolateral uterus.
- Ovaries appear as round or ellipsoid structures with a hyperechoic rim and often multiple, cyst-like ovarian follicles—often described as a "chocolate chip cookie."

- Short-axis: Ovaries can sometimes be seen in the same plane as the superior lateral portion of the uterus.
  - Alternatively, angle the beam toward the right or left shoulder to view the respective adnexal structures.
- Long-axis: From starting position slide probe right or left to look for the corresponding ovary.
  - Alternatively, angle beam toward the contralateral adnexa (e.g., look left from the right side) to utilize the bladder as a window.

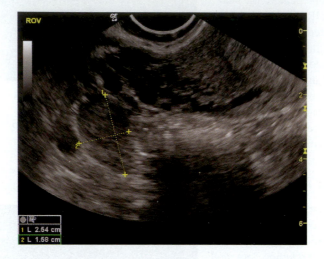

PATHOLOGY

- Subchorionic hemorrhage (*): Anechoic stripe seen between the gestational sac and the myometrium.

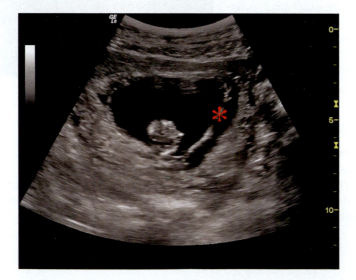

- Absence of cardiac motion in an embryo >7–8 weeks or 10 mm in length (TA) is consistent with fetal demise.
- Suggestive of extrauterine pregnancy (EP): No IUP seen plus pelvic masses outside the uterus, or eccentrically located uterine mass, free fluid (*) in the pelvis or abdomen.

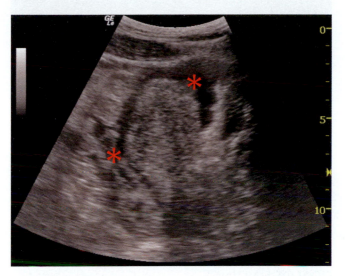

- Definite EP: Pregnancy-related structures/FHR seen outside the uterus.
- Interstitial pregnancy (*): Eccentrically located IUP but has <8 mm of surrounding myometrium at its thinnest point.

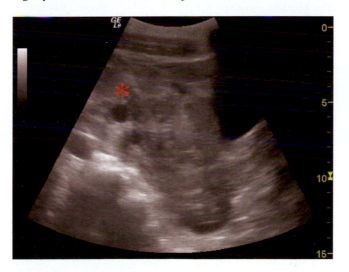

- Molar pregnancy (*): Mass of varying size within the uterus with multiple hypoechoic internal vesicles creating a snowstorm or bag of grapes appearance. Serum HCG usually markedly elevated.

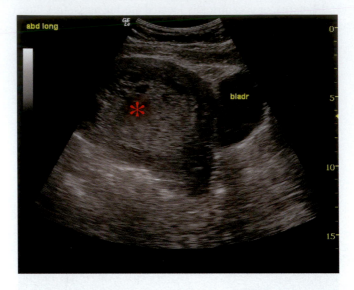

INTEGRATION OF FINDINGS

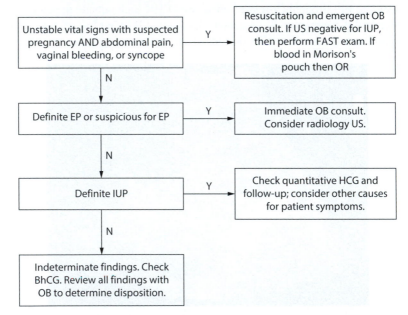

SPECIAL CONSIDERATIONS

- In the unstable female patient of child-bearing age without trauma, an empty uterus and blood in Morison's pouch is a ruptured ectopic pregnancy requiring emergent OB/GYN evaluation and management.
- The risk of heterotopic pregnancy in the general population is very low, but increases to as high as 1 in 4000 in women on fertility drugs.

8 Appendicitis

Frances Russell and John Bailitz

INDICATIONS

- Rule in suspected appendicitis in pediatric, pregnant, and thin adult patients[1]

IMAGE ACQUISITION AND INTERPRETATION

EQUIPMENT

- High-frequency linear probe for thin and pediatric patients, or convex transducer for larger patients

PREPARATION

- Place the patient in supine position with the knees bent to relax the abdomen.
- Administer small doses of pain medications prior to the performance of the ultrasound exam to reduce patient discomfort during the ultrasound exam.
- Perform ultrasound prior to administration of oral contrast.

TECHNIQUE

TRANSDUCER POSITION

- Begin by asking the patient to identify with one finger the site of maximal pain. Confirm this as the site of maximal tenderness with gentle palpation. Place the probe directly over the identified site.
- Apply constant graded compression over this area to displace air within the bowel that may be obscuring the view of the appendix.

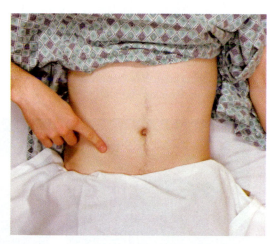

---

[1] Refer to Chapter 14 for the pediatric assessment for appendicitis.

- Scan the area in both the transverse and longitudinal planes.
- When the appendix is not readily visualized, survey the right lower quadrant by visualizing the iliac vessels from the aortic bifurcation to the inguinal ligament. The appendix is often anterior to the external iliac vessel.

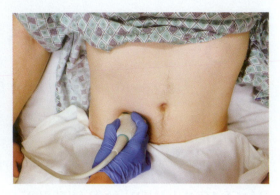

Normal Anatomy

- The appendix (*) is a compressible, finger-like structure, with a maximal outer diameter less than 6 mm and subtle peristalsis. May be difficult to visualize when normal.

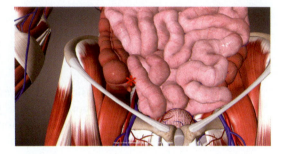

Pathology

- Appendicitis (*)
  - Non-compressible target or bull's-eye appearing structure in short axis
  - Diameter greater than 6 mm
  - Lack of peristalsis
  - Increased color flow
- An appendicolith is visualized as a hyperechoic structure within the appendix with acoustic shadowing.

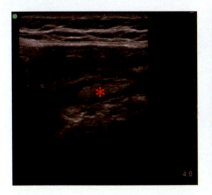

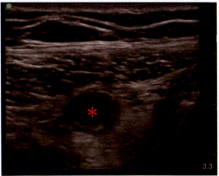

- Perforated appendicitis: Appendix decompresses and may be harder to visualize if a periappendiceal abscess has not yet formed.
- Specificity of POCS for appendicitis is high but the sensitivity is low. Negative findings do not rule out appendicitis.

INTEGRATION OF FINDINGS

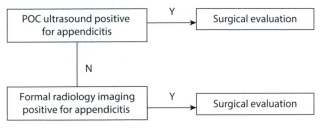

SPECIAL CONSIDERATIONS

- Ultrasound is often the initial imaging modality of choice for pediatric, pregnant, and thin patients due to its safety profile.

9 Ocular Ultrasound

Dasia Esener

INDICATIONS

- Assess vision loss or impairment
- Evaluate eye trauma

IMAGE ACQUISITION AND INTERPRETATION

EQUIPMENT

- High frequency linear probe
- High frequency endocavity probe

PREPARATION

- Sterile adhesive for eye protection
- Ultrasound gel

STEPS

1. Identify normal structures.
2. Identify abnormal structures and foreign bodies.

SONOGRAPHIC LANDMARKS

1. Cornea
2. Anterior chamber
3. Pupil
4. Ciliary body
5. Posterior chamber
6. Lens artifact
7. Vitreous
8. Retina
9. Optic nerve

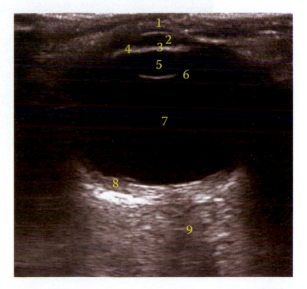

Step 1: Identify normal structures

- Place probe in transverse orientation over the center of the eye with probe indicator pointing temporally.[1]
- Rest the wrist or little finger on the patient's face to avoid unnecessary pressure on eye.
- Identify the lens, vitreous, and retina.
- Note that the retina is hyperechoic and tethered at the optic nerve; the vitreous is anechoic.
- Have patient move eye left, right, up, and down.
- Change probe positioning to the sagittal orientation and repeat the exam.
- Evaluate both the affected and non-affected eye.

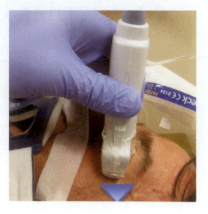

Step 2: Identify abnormal structures and foreign bodies

- Have the patient look in all four directions while observing movement within the globe such as vitreous hemorrhage, foreign bodies, or detached retina.
- Foreign body (*).

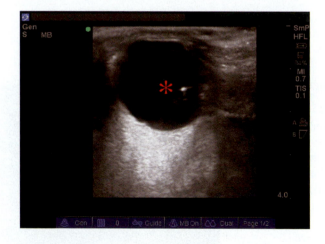

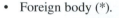

[1] The macula is temporal to the optic nerve; placing the probe indicator temporally ensures that the macula is always on the side of the indicator on the screen. This is important when evaluating retinal pathology.

- Ocular lymphoma (*).

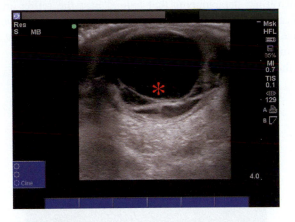

- Retinal detachment (*).

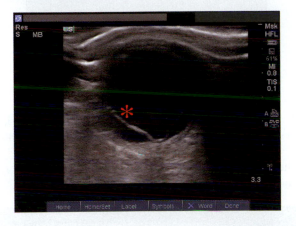

- Note when the retina detaches, a thin, hyperechoic membrane floats freely in the vitreous (*).

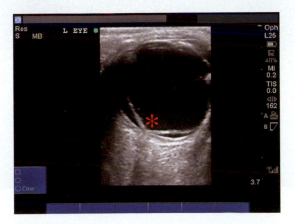

- Evaluate whether the detached retina extends beyond the macula.
- Note that retinal detachments that extend past the retina are considered "macula off" and will have central vision abnormalities on eye exam.
- Recognize that retina is tethered to the optic nerve posteriorly and remains tethered in retinal detachments.
- Vitreous hemorrhage (*).

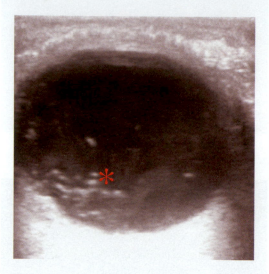

- Note that vitreous hemorrhage appears as mobile vitreous opacities.
- Differentiating vitreous hemorrhage from other vitreous pathology can be difficult.
- Vitreous hemorrhage will change in echogenicity as it ages, forming layers.
- Lens dislocation (*).

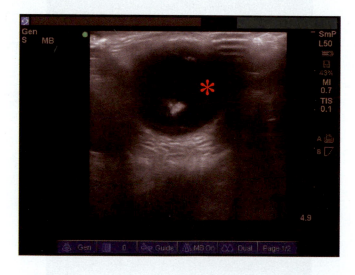

- Note that lens dislocation will appear as an oval structure within the vitreous and a void between the iris on either side.
- Partial dislocations can be difficult to diagnose sonographically because the lens is usually in the correct position.
- Complete dislocations are obvious due to the lens being found in the vitreous.
- Globe rupture (*).

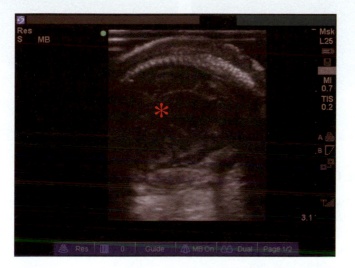

- Recognize destruction of globe shape and sonographic landmarks.
- Optic nerve sheath diameter. Optic nerve diameter may be measured if there is concern for elevated ICP. The optic nerve sheath diameter should be measured 3 mm from the globe. Normally the diameter should be less than 5 mm.
- Measure 3 mm vertically from the globe along optic nerve trajectory.
- Measure the optic nerve sheath diameter at this point.

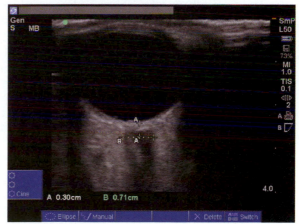

- Note bulging of the optic disc (*) into the vitreous can be seen with increased ICP/papilledema.

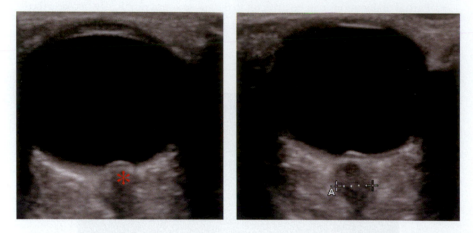

SPECIAL CONSIDERATIONS

- Consensual papillary response can be demonstrated in patients by exposing uninvolved eye to light and evoking iris constriction under ultrasound visualization.
- Place probe indicator temporally so that the macula is always on the side of the screen indicator.
- Use the optic nerve as a landmark when evaluating the retina.
- Use extreme caution when evaluating patients with potential globe rupture; use copious amounts of gel and do not place unnecessary pressure on the eye.
- Use of an adhesive dressing on a closed eye increases patient comfort and prevents gel from entering eye. Be sure to lay it flush over the eye and push out underlying air bubbles.

10 Soft Tissue Procedures

Mikaela Chilstrom

INDICATIONS

- Differentiate normal tissue from edema, infection, and focal fluid collections
- Determine the nature and extent of soft tissue fluid collections (abscess, cyst, lipoma)
- Identify and localize foreign bodies

IMAGE ACQUISITION AND INTERPRETATION

EQUIPMENT

- High-frequency linear probe
- Endocavity probe for peritonsillar abscesses

PREPARATION

- Apply copious gel to affected areas.
- Consider water bath or standoff pads (commercial or IV bags) to minimize discomfort from probe pressure.
- Use sterile technique with probe cover or large sterile adhesive if using dynamic scanning technique.

SOFT TISSUE INFECTION

- Review normal regional anatomy.
- Evaluate area of suspected pathology.
- Locate and mark the optimal incision site.

Step 1: Review normal regional anatomy

- Scan contralateral side or unaffected nearby areas in longitudinal and transverse planes.
- Specifically identify normal dermis, subcutaneous tissue, facial planes, muscle, tendons, ligaments, nerves, and vessels.

Step 2: Evaluate areas of suspected pathology

- Scan affected areas in two planes.
- Edema: Hypoechoic areas of anechoic fluid separate the subcutaneous tissue creating a "cobblestone" appearance. May be seen in both cellulitis and edema due to other causes.
- Cellulitis: Skin and soft tissue will appear hyperechoic with blurring or even loss of normal soft tissue landmarks.

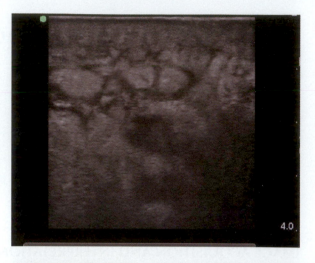

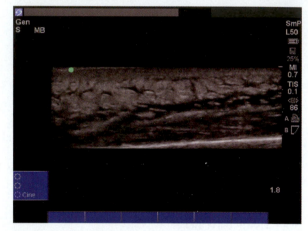

Abscess

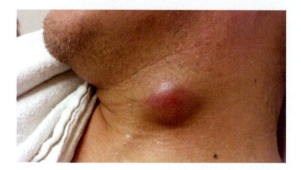

- Anechoic to mixed echogenic fluid collections surrounded by an often irregular border of hyperechoic tissue (*).
- Depending on age and cause, abscess cavity may be round or irregular, which may destroy the fascial planes.
- Internal echoes may result from septations or gas.
- Apply gentle pressure with probe to move purulent material within abscess.
- Identify nearby ligaments, tendons, nerves, lymph nodes, and vessels to avoid during incision and drainage.
- Color flow Doppler can assist in defining vascular structures.

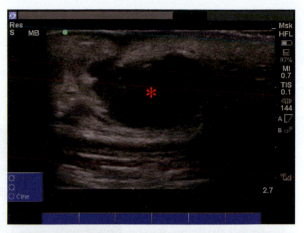

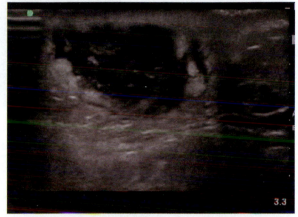

Step 3: Mark incision site

- Estimate the length, width, and depth of a fluid collection.
- The ideal incision site is the most superficial central area of the abscess.
- Mark this area with hash marks in two perpendicular planes to define anesthetic deposition and incision site.

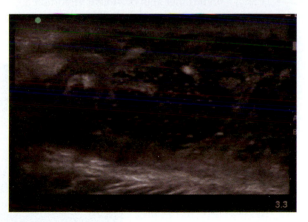

FOREIGN BODY

- Scan the area of interest to localize the foreign body.
- Measure the size and depth of the foreign body in two planes.
- Localize the foreign body sonographically with a needle.
- Extract foreign body.

Step 1: Localize the foreign body

- Place the probe over the area of interest.
- Foreign bodies will generally appear as hyperechoic structures with posterior acoustic shadowing. Metallic structures may create reverberation or comet tail artifacts.
- Retained or infected foreign bodies may be surrounded by hypoechoic fluid.

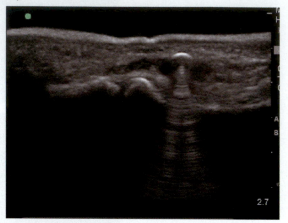

Step 2: Measure the size and depth of the foreign body

- Measure the length and width of the foreign body in two dimensions.
- Determine the depth of the foreign body.
- Identify other pertinent nearby structures tendons, ligaments, bones, nerves, lymph nodes, and vessels.
- Foreign bodies that abut or violate important adjacent structures, or are deeply imbedded in soft tissue, should be referred to a specialist for removal.

Step 3: Localize the foreign body with needle(s)

- Visualize the foreign body in long axis with the probe parallel to the foreign body.
- Anesthetize overlying skin and soft tissue.
- Advance two different needles under real time in plane visualization to delineate the opposite ends of the foreign body.

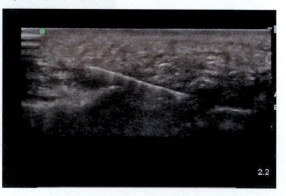

Step 4: Remove foreign body

- Anesthetize the region between the two needles and make an incision between the two needles (directly above the foreign body). Cut down to the foreign body and extract using forceps or hemostat.
- Alternatively, make an incision and remove over the most superficial portion of the foreign body.

SPECIAL CONSIDERATIONS

- Foreign bodies that are deeply imbedded in soft tissue or abut or violate vital adjacent structures are not appropriate for removal in the emergency department. Refer to a specialist for definitive removal.
- Even in difficult cases, ultrasound may be helpful for identification of foreign bodies and proper referral.
- Instruct patients that a foreign body may still be present despite a negative ultrasound evaluation. Provide appropriate wound care and follow-up.

11 Musculoskeletal

Joy English and Mikaela Chilstrom

INDICATIONS

- Evaluate for suspected tendon trauma or inflammation
- Assess for the presence of subtle fractures or dislocation

TENDON ULTRASOUND

IMAGE ACQUISITION AND INTERPRETATION

EQUIPMENT

- High frequency linear probe
- Water baths and standoff pads (small IV bags) are helpful to minimize discomfort when visualizing superficial structures
- Low frequency curvilinear probe may better visualize large joints and deeper structures

PREPARATION

- Position patient in the most comfortable position that allows access to the affected area.

RECOMMENDED VIEWS

1. Begin by visualizing the contralateral or nearby unaffected tendons in both the transverse and longitudinal axis.
2. Evaluate the affected tendon next in both the transverse and longitudinal axis.

TRANSDUCER PLACEMENT

- Place the probe in axial orientation over the tendon to obtain a short axis view.
- Ensure that the probe is situated exactly 90 degrees to the skin surface.

- Tendons, muscle, and nerves exhibit the property of anisotropy (*). The fibrillar arrangement of these structures will appear hyperechoic when the ultrasound beam is exactly perpendicular to the fibers, but hypoechoic at other angles.

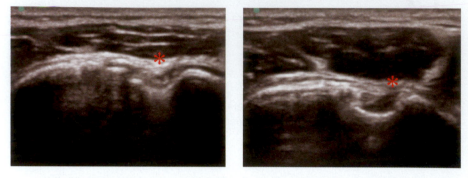

- Rotate the probe 90 degrees to obtain a long axis view of the tendon.

NORMAL ANATOMY

- Tendons: Tightly packed fascicles of parallel collagen fibers.
- Short axis: Hyperechoic structures with hypoechoic dots.
- Longitudinal axis: Hyperechoic lines (*) closely arranged in a fibrillar arrangement.
- Variable cross-sectional shape: The long head of the biceps tendon is round, the Achilles tendon oval, and the patellar tendon rectangular.

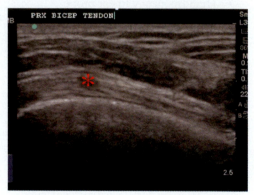

PATHOLOGY

- Full tendon tear: Complete disruption of fibrillar architecture, no proximal tendon movement with passive motion.
- Partial tendon tear: Hypoechoic area within the normal tendon architecture.
- Tenosynovitis: Tendon thickening and tendon sheath widening. Loss of normal tendon fibrillar architecture. Variable amount of anechoic fluid collection surrounding tendon (*).

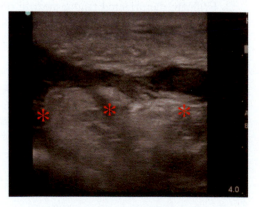

SPECIAL CONSIDERATIONS

- Do not mistake anisotropy for pathology. If there is a hypoechoic area of tendon, rock the transducer end to end in the long axis to change the angle of the ultrasound beam. Disappearance of the hypoechoic area indicates anisotropy. A persistent hypoechoic defect represents tendon pathology.

FRACTURE DIAGNOSIS

INDICATIONS

- Evaluate for suspected long bone fracture. This is then especially helpful in the pediatric population, out-of-hospital medicine, and remote medicine including international, military, and tactical medicine.
- Assess for subtle bone trauma where plain radiographs may be nondiagnostic or normal (rib fractures).
- Detect early stress fractures.

IMAGE ACQUISITION AND INTERPRETATION

EQUIPMENT

- Linear 10–15 Mhz provides excellent near-field resolution for superficial structures.
- Curvilinear 3–5 Mhz transducer improves visualization of bones located >6 cm deep to the surface but sacrifices near-field resolution.
- Apply generous amount of gel to improve surface contact over painful areas. Use a standoff pad or water bath if appropriate contact cannot be maintained.

PREPARATION

- Place the patient in a position of comfort that also allows for adequate ultrasound examination.
- Medication for pain will almost always be necessary, as the main area of focus will be directly over the suspected fracture site.

RECOMMENDED VIEWS

1. Begin by visualizing the contralateral or nearby unaffected bone in both the transverse and longitudinal axis, from an anterior and posterior approach.
2. Then visualize the affected bone in both the transverse and longitudinal axis as well as the anterior and posterior planes.

TRANSDUCER PLACEMENT

- Place the probe directly over the suspected site of fracture. Move slowly and systematically in the long axis and then the short axis. Then move the probe in the anterior/posterior axis systematically as above.

NORMAL ANATOMY

- Bones appear as a bright white line without disruption. The immediate overlying soft tissue should appear homogenous along the entire length of the bone.
- Closely evaluate the physis in children, which represents a normal disruption of the cortex.

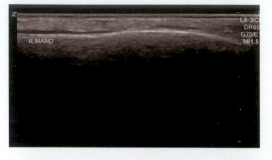

PATHOLOGY

- Fractures (*) appear as an unexpected discontinuity of the cortex.

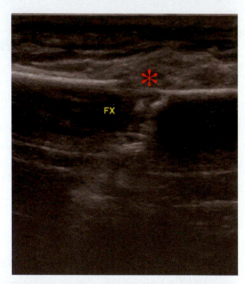

- A hematoma (*) may occur in the surrounding soft tissues and will appear as a hypoechoic area close to the bone.
- Heterogeneity of the overlying soft tissue may represent a subtle fracture. In children with open physis it may represent a Salter–Harris type I fracture.

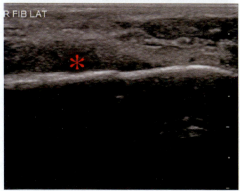

SPECIAL CONSIDERATIONS

- Ultrasound identifies Salter–Harris I fractures with higher sensitivity than plain radiographs by identifying hematoma formation and heterogeneity of overlying soft tissues. Obtain plain radiographs, splint, and refer for further evaluation.

12 Lower Extremity Deep Vein Thrombosis

Nadim Hafez

INDICATIONS

- Evaluate lower extremity pain or swelling suggestive of deep venous thrombosis (DVT)
- Detect other causes of leg pain and swelling such as ruptured Baker cyst, abscess, or cellulitis (see Chapter 10, "Soft Tissue Procedures")

IMAGE ACQUISITION AND INTERPRETATION

EQUIPMENT

- High frequency linear probe (8–12 MHz)
- Curvilinear probe (3–6 MHz) for obese patients

PREPARATION

- Place patient in the supine position with the head of the bed elevated 30 degrees, hip slightly abducted and externally rotated, and knee flexed.
- Place line of gel over the anticipated course of vessel to facilitate "stepping down the leg" without the need to constantly reapply gel to the probe.
- Ask the patient or an assistant to retract the abdominal pannus if needed to properly visualize the inguinal area while keeping the probe perpendicular to vessel.

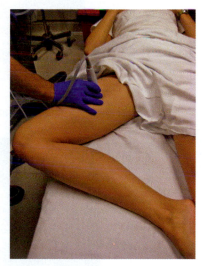

RECOMMENDED VIEWS

1. Femoral vein
   a. Common femoral artery (CFA) and common femoral vein (CFV)
   b. CFV and greater saphenous vein (GSV)
   c. Bifurcation of CFV into superficial femoral vein (SFV) and deep femoral vein (DFV)

2. Popliteal vein
   a. Proximal popliteal vein
   b. Distal popliteal vein

FEMORAL VEIN

TRANSDUCER PLACEMENT

- Place the transducer at the inguinal ligament in the transverse plane with the indicator pointing toward the patient's right.

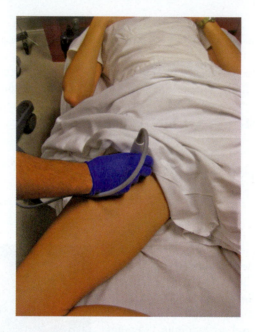

- Visualize the CFV and GSV junction and CFA (*).

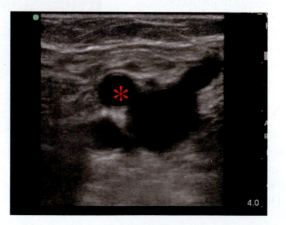

- Step down the leg by lifting the probe and moving distally in 1 cm increments, then compressing again. Visualize the GSV entering the CFV.
- Continue down the leg until the CFV bifurcates into the SFV and DFV. The majority of FV DVTs are between the inguinal ligament and the bifurcation.

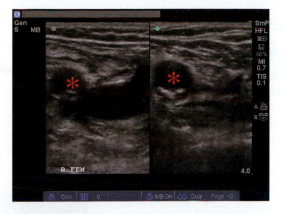

- At each step, if no thrombus is visualized, then compress the anterior and posterior walls of the vein.
- A normal vein will completely compress without significant distortion of the adjacent artery.

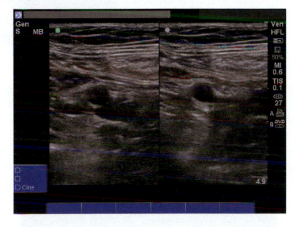

NORMAL ANATOMY

- Common femoral vein (CFV): From caudad to cephalad in the direction of venous flow:
  - The SFV and DFV join to form the CFV. The term SFV must not be mistaken for a superficial vein; the SFV is a deep vein.
  - The CFV is joined by the greater saphenous vein just caudad to the inguinal ligament.
  - The CFV continues cephalad to become the external iliac vein at the inguinal ligament.

- Common femoral artery (CFA): From cephalad to caudad in the direction of arterial flow:
  - Bifurcates into superficial and deep femoral artery (SFA and DFA) just below the inguinal ligament.

POPLITEAL VEIN

TRANSDUCER PLACEMENT

- Place the transducer in the middle of the popliteal fossa in the transverse plane to identify the popliteal artery (PA) and popliteal vein (PV).
- Step cephalad to visualize the proximal PV and PA.
- Then slowly step caudad to visualize the PV through the trifurcation.

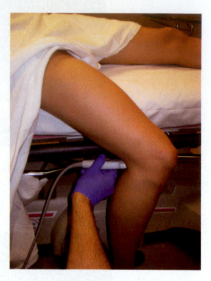

NORMAL ANATOMY

- The PV arises from the anterior tibial, posterior tibial, and peroneal veins in the calf, runs superficial to the PA through the popliteal fossa, then runs cephalad above the knee to become the SFV.

PATHOLOGY

- The majority of DVTs occur in the CFV or SFV within the proximal 1/3 of the thigh, or in the popliteal fossa. Neither the middle 1/3 of the thigh, nor the DFV need to be visualized routinely.
- Inability to compress the vein completely without significant deformation of the artery warrants appropriate therapy.
- CFA (*) with CFV underneath before compression (left) and after compression (right). Lack of compression on right denotes presence of DVT.

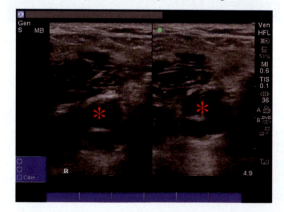

- Popliteal vein is easily compressible.
- If the artery collapses under pressure but the vein does not, this is highly indicative of a DVT.

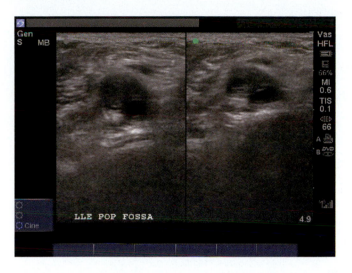

INTEGRATION OF FINDINGS

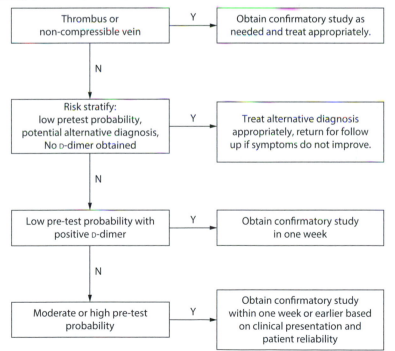

13 Vascular Access

Dasia Esener

PERIPHERAL ACCESS

INDICATIONS

- Improve visualization of vascular landmarks and surrounding structures in patients when blind IV placement is difficult
- Increase accuracy and success of IV placement to any peripheral vein

EQUIPMENT

- High frequency linear probe
- Long IV catheter (preferably 2–2.5 inches, 18–22 gauge)
- Marking pen if using static method
- Sterile adhesive dressing

PERIPHERAL LINE PLACEMENT

PREPARATION

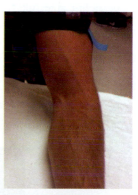

- Apply a tourniquet to the extremity before gathering supplies.
- Place the ultrasound screen within the direct line of site.
- Pre-scan the entire area to visualize vascular landmarks and surrounding structures.
- Apply gel and cover the end of the probe with a sterile adhesive dressing.
- Dynamic technique is preferred for direct real-time visualization.
- Static technique can be used to locate the vessel prior to the standard traditional blind cannulation. A marking pen may be used to mark the proximal and distal portions of the vessel. The patient's position must not be changed after marking.

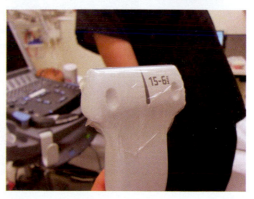

- Visualization and cannulation in the transverse plane localizes the target vessel in relation to nearby structures, reducing the risk of inadvertent puncture.
- The sagittal plane provides real-time direct visualization of the entire needle along the path to the target vessel.

STEPS FOR PERIPHERAL LINE PLACEMENT

1. Identify the vessel.
2. Cannulate the vessel.
3. Confirm placement.

Step 1: Identify the vessel

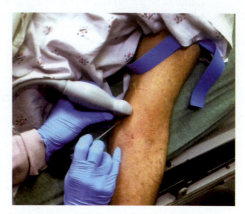

- Place the probe in the transverse orientation, just medial and proximal to the antecubital fossa. Use minimal pressure to avoid collapsing superficial veins.
- Scan the vessel in both the transverse and sagittal plane to accurately determine vessel patency, depth, size, and trajectory.
- Higher success rates are achieved with veins between 3 mm–1 cm deep and at least 3 mm in diameter.

Basilic Vein

- Runs superficially along the medial aspect of the arm in the groove between the biceps and triceps.

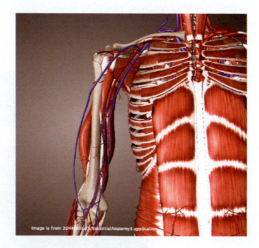

Image is from 3D4Medical's EssentialAnatomy3 application

Cephalic Vein
- Runs superficially along the anterolateral aspect of arm.

Deep Brachial Veins
- The medial and lateral branches of the deep brachial vein run on either side of the brachial artery. The artery will be pulsatile and more difficult to collapse with pressure.
- The deeper brachial vein has a higher risk of infiltration and may result in paresthesias due to irritation of the adjacent median nerve.

Step 2: Cannulate vessel

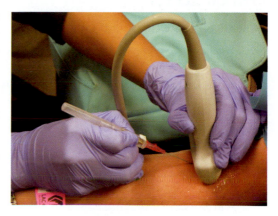

- With your non-dominant hand, hold probe in transverse orientation perpendicular to the vessel.
- Locate and center the vessel on the screen.
- Use your non-dominant hand to hold the probe while you puncture the skin just distal to the center of the probe and advance a few millimeters at a 45-degree angle to the vessel.
- Visualize the needle tip in the tissue. As the needle tip is advanced, slide the probe proximal to the puncture site to maintain direct visualization of the needle tip. For a typical vein that is 1 cm deep, venous puncture will occur at a cannula length of about 1.4 cm when inserting the needle at this 45-degree angle. This will increase with a deeper vessel or shallower angle.
- Centering the vessel on the screen ensures that the vessel is positioned along the middle of the probe.
- Puncture the superficial wall and advance the needle 1 mm further to ensure catheter is within the vessel. The catheter will advance easily once in lumen.
- If the catheter does not advance easily or the patient experiences significant discomfort, then readjust the catheter position.
- Obtaining a flash, then losing blood return indicates that the needle tip has likely advanced beyond the vessel lumen. Slowly withdraw the needle under ultrasound guidance until the needle lies within the lumen and blood return is again noted.
- The sagittal approach can also be attempted when the vessel is very straight and superficial. Use caution however, when arteries or nerves are within close proximity.

Step 3: Confirm placement

- Easy deployment of the catheter over the needle with blood return initially confirms placement.
- Next, visualize the catheter in the vessel using the longitudinal or transverse approach to the vessel. Keep the tourniquet on to distend the vessel and improve visualization of the catheter within the lumen.
- If the vessel is difficult to visualize, briefly shake a syringe of saline, flush, and watch the agitated saline go through into the lumen of the vein with ultrasound.

CENTRAL ACCESS

INDICATIONS FOR ULTRASOUND GUIDANCE

- Improve accuracy, first-pass cannulation rate, patient satisfaction, and success of central IV placement
- Decrease rate of arterial and nerve puncture, failed cannulation, number of attempts

EQUIPMENT

- High frequency linear probe
- Sterile probe cover in addition to standard sterile central line kit, gown, and gloves

PREPARATION

- Position machine and patient so that the insertion site is directly between the sonographer and the screen.
- Pre-scan along the length of the entire vessel in both transverse and sagittal planes to determine patency, depth, size, and trajectory prior to getting sterile.
- Apply a copious amount of gel to the ultrasound probe.
- Put on sterile gloves and gown. Encase probe within a sterile probe cover by placing hand inside of the probe cover and grabbing the probe, which is in an upright position on the ultrasound cart, and pulling the sterile sheath down over the probe cord.
- Press finger on face of probe to remove air bubbles between probe cover and underlying gel, and place sterile rubber bands over probe cover to attach it to probe.
- Lay sterile probe on sterile field covering patient. Place a small amount of sterile ultrasound gel on the sterile field.

STEPS FOR CENTRAL INTERNAL JUGULAR LINE PLACEMENT

1. Identify vessel
2. Cannulate vessel
3. Confirm placement

Step 1: Identify vessel

- Place a small amount of sterile gel on the now-sterile probe. After identifying traditional anatomic landmarks, again scan along the length of the vessel in both transverse and sagittal planes to confirm patency, depth, size, and trajectory of the target vessel.
- Note the location of the artery, important nearby neurovascular structures, and apex of the lung.
- Note that the vein will compress easily and the artery will not.
- Identify a skin puncture site where the vein is lateral to the nearby artery.

Step 2: Cannulate vessel

- With your non-dominant hand, hold probe in transverse orientation perpendicular to the vessel (preferably with the probe indicator to your left). Locate and then center the vessel on the screen.
- With your dominant hand, puncture the skin just distal to the center of the probe and advance a few millimeters at a 45-degree angle to the vessel.
- Visualize the needle tip in the tissue. As the needle tip is advanced, slide the probe away from the puncture site to maintain direct visualization of the needle tip.
- For a typical vein that is 1 cm deep, puncture will occur at a cannula length of about 1.4 cm when inserting the needle at this 45-degree angle. This will increase with a deeper vessel or shallower angle.
- Puncture the superficial wall and advance the needle 1 mm further to ensure catheter is within the vessel. The catheter will advance easily once in lumen.
- If the catheter does not advance easily or the patient experiences significant discomfort, then readjust the catheter position.
- Obtaining a flash, then losing blood return indicates that the needle tip has likely advanced beyond the vessel lumen. Slowly withdraw the needle under ultrasound guidance until the needle lies within the lumen and blood return is again noted.
- To re-direct the needle trajectory, pull the needle almost entirely back then re-advance in the appropriate direction to avoid injury.

Step 3: Confirm placement

- Easy deployment of the catheter over the needle with blood return initially confirms placement.

- Next, visualize the catheter in the vessel (*) using the sagittal (easier) or transverse (harder) approach of the vessel. Keep the tourniquet on to distend the vessel and improve visualization of the catheter within the lumen.

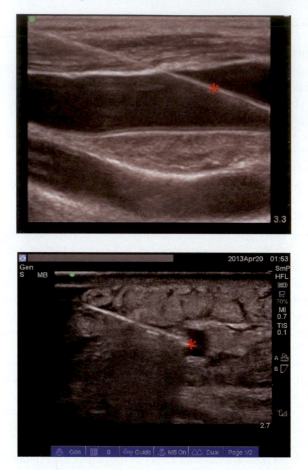

- When difficult to visualize, briefly shake a saline syringe, flush, and watch the agitated saline go into the lumen of the vein or into the heart.

SPECIAL CONSIDERATIONS

- Arterial lines can be placed in a similar method as venous lines. Note that the artery is thicker walled, and spasms with compression.
- With sufficient experience, upper arm peripheral IVs are invaluable in sick children. For infants and toddlers, use higher-gauge shorter catheters. However, when possible use catheters at least 1.25 inches in length to facilitate ultrasound visualization.

14 Pediatric

Russ Horowitz

INDICATIONS

- Evaluate for intussusception, pyloric stenosis, appendicitis, and fractures
- Streamline care to reduce the need for other imaging

INTUSSUSCEPTION

IMAGE ACQUISITION AND INTERPRETATION

EQUIPMENT

- High frequency linear probe

PREPARATION

- Ensure that the child is comfortable.
- Place child in the supine position on the bed or on a caregiver's lap.
- Warm gel to maximize patient comfort.

TRANSDUCER PLACEMENT

- Begin in right lower quadrant to visualize cecum, which is bordered laterally by pelvic brim (hyperechoic oblique line with posterior shadowing), and appears as a wide tubular structure in the sagittal plane filled with hypoechoic fluid and hyperechoic air bubbles.
- Place probe in transverse plane and proceed cephalad to visualize the entire ascending colon.
- Once the liver is visualized, rotate probe 90 degrees into the sagittal plane with the indicator pointing toward the child's head and proceed to splenic flexure.

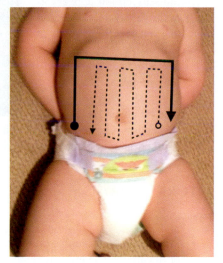

- Rotate probe 90 degrees into the transverse plane, proceed caudally, and complete the survey of the descending colon.
- To completely visualize the bowel, perform a systemic evaluation of the entire abdomen including the small intestine.
- Use graded compression (slow steady pressure) to push gas out of view to better image the bowel.

Normal Anatomy

- Normal bowel: Appears as a mix of reverberating horizontal hyperechoic lines similar to the A-lines seen on the pleura views of the lung, muscular bowel wall with visible villi, and hyperechoic air bubbles.
- Bowel peristalsis: Seen as movement of hyperechoic air bubbles and intestinal contents.

Pathology

- Intussusception: Most commonly occurs at the ileocolic junction and is often seen at the hepatic flexure.
- In cross-section (*), intussusception appears as concentric rings commonly referred to as the pseudokidney sign, target sign, or bull's-eye sign.
- In the longitudinal plane, intussusception appears as multiple layers on top of one another, or a stack of pancakes.
- Intussuscepted bowel will have no peristalsis.
- Large stools within colon may be mistaken for intussusception. Graded compression may be used to advance the stool and differentiate it from true intussusception.

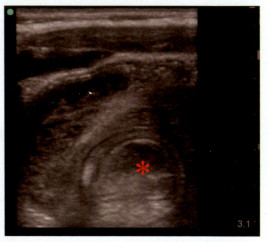

PYLORIC STENOSIS

Preparation

- Place child in the supine or in the right lateral decubitus position on the bed, or in caregiver's lap.
- A small amount of fluid may be fed to the child to distend the stomach and improve visualization of the pylorus and fluid passage.

TRANSDUCER PLACEMENT

- Begin with the probe in the epigastrium just medial to the medial border of the liver.
- Place the probe in the sagittal plane to visualize the pylorus along its length and in the transverse plane to visualize it in cross section.

NORMAL ANATOMY

- The pylorus is bordered laterally by the liver and gallbladder (*) and medially and superiorly by the stomach (*).
- A normal pylorus measures less than 15 mm in length and less than 3 mm in thickness.
- Fluid is seen traversing the pylorus and entering the duodenum.

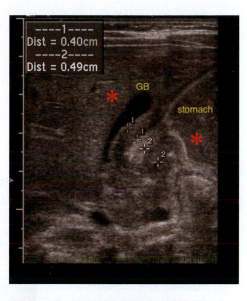

PATHOLOGY

Both pictures from patient with pyloric stenosis.

- Pyloric stenosis: No fluid is seen passing through the pylorus.
- Greater than 15 mm in length and 3 mm in thickness.

SPECIAL CONSIDERATIONS

- Overdistention of the stomach will shift the pylorus posteriorly and impair visualization.
- Overlying bowel gas may obscure visualization.

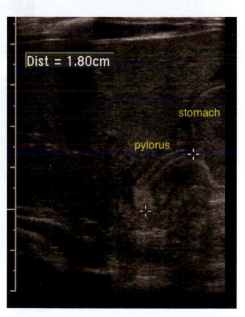

APPENDICITIS

EQUIPMENT

- High-frequency linear probe for thinner patients
- Lower frequency curvilinear probe for larger patients

PREPARATION

- Place child in supine position on the bed or a caregiver's lap.
- Use of parenteral pain control is essential for patient comfort.
- Minimize probe pressure to reduce patient discomfort.

TRANSDUCER PLACEMENT

- Begin with probe in right lower quadrant in the area of McBurney's point.
- Self-localization: Place probe in point of maximal tenderness.

NORMAL ANATOMY

- Identify appendix by locating neighboring structures. Illiac vessels are medial. The psoas muscle (striated appearance) often lies deep to appendix. The appendix protrudes from the medial edge of the cecum.
- A non-visualized appendix may be retrocecal.
- Use the non-imaging hand to apply pressure to the flank to bring appendix into view.

PATHOLOGY: APPENDICITIS

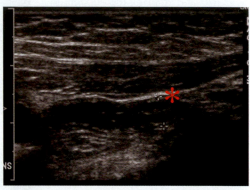

- A blind loop structure (*) (without peristalsis)
- >6 mm in thickness
- Non-compressible
- Hyperemic on color flow
- Fecalith (may or may not shadow)

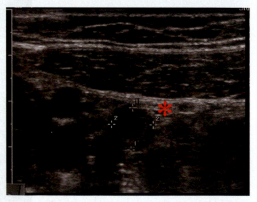

- Target or bull's-eye appearance in cross section (*)

SPECIAL CONSIDERATIONS

- Apply direct pressure to appendix to assess compressibility.
- Use graded compression to push overlying bowel gas out of the way.
- Obese patients make visualization difficult.
- A non-visualized appendix is a nondiagnostic study.
- Ruptured appendicitis will show surrounding hypoechoic fluid or abscess.
- Necrotic appendix will not have a hyperemic appearance, but instead have no flow.

FRACTURES

EQUIPMENT

- High frequency linear probe
- Standoff pad or water bath based on site of suspected fracture
- Copious gel to allow the probe to float over the bone and eliminate contact associated pain

PREPARATION

- Maintain patient in position of comfort to reduce pain.
- Use of copious pain control is essential.
- Minimize probe pressure to reduce pain and discomfort.

TRANSDUCER PLACEMENT

- Orient probe marker toward distal end of bone of interest.
- Scan the bone in multiple planes.

NORMAL ANATOMY

- Normal bone appears as a continuous hyperechoic line.
- Growth plates appear as an anechoic space between the distal metaphysis and epiphysis.
- The distal metaphysis and proximal epiphysis have a gentle curve inward (*) toward the growth plate. Do not confuse these with fracture sites.

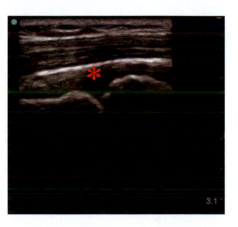

PATHOLOGY

- A fracture (*) is defined sonographically as a visible cortical bone disruption or step-off, with or without overlying hematoma.

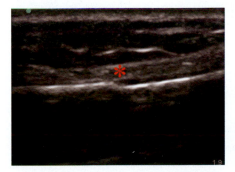 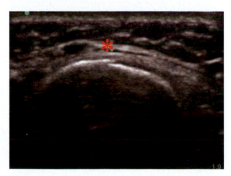

15 Abdominal Procedures

John Lemos

INDICATIONS

- To confirm the presence of ascites and a fluid pocket large enough to safely access the peritoneum
- To identify and avoid overlying vascular structures and surrounding abdominal organs

IMAGE ACQUISITION AND INTERPRETATION

EQUIPMENT

- Curvilinear probe
- Sterile probe cover and gel for dynamic scanning
- Marking pen for static scanning
- Paracentesis supplies

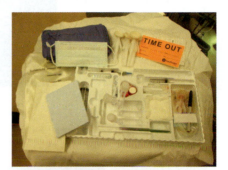

PREPARATION

- Position the patient in slight reverse Trendelenburg and a lateral decubitus position to allow fluid to accumulate in the lower abdomen on one side.
- Consider having the patient void, or place a Foley catheter to empty the bladder prior to the procedure.
- Pre-scan the patient prior to sterile setup to confirm the presence of ascites. Ascites will appear as anechoic fluid surrounding the abdominal organs. Loops of bowel will be seen floating in the fluid.

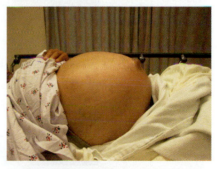

STEPS

1. Identify the best pocket of fluid.
2. Confirm the absence of overlying vascular structures.

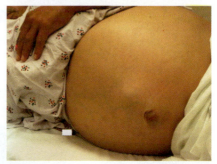

3. Calculate the depth of the fluid pocket from the skin surface and center the probe.
4. Insert needle and aspirate fluid.

Step 1: Identify the best pocket of fluid

- Place probe on patient in one of the lower quadrants of the abdomen approximately 4 cm superior and medial to the anterior superior iliac spine (ASIS).

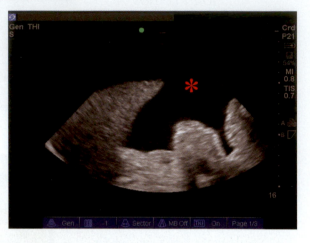

- Use the ultrasound to confirm that the bladder is empty and is not in the projected pathway of your needle. The bladder will appear as a hypoechoic fluid-filled structure with a bright wall separating it from the surrounding ascites.
- Visualize the largest pocket of fluid as identified.

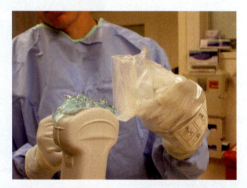

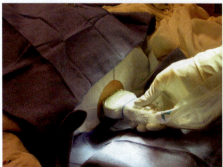

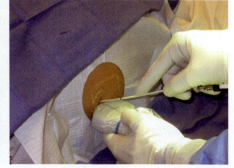

Step 2: Confirm the absence of overlying vasculature

- Decrease depth on the screen to visualize vasculature structures, such as the inferior epigastric arteries that lie close to the abdominal wall surface.

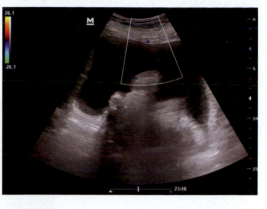

- Ensure that probe application on patient is not compressing or obscuring the vasculature.
- Consider performing the procedure in the midline or lower laterally to avoid the inferior epigastric arteries.

Step 3: Calculate the depth of the fluid pocket and center the probe

- Calculate the depth of the fluid pocket by using the markers at the side of the ultrasound screen.

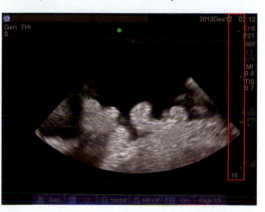

- Center the probe so that the largest area of fluid is in the middle of the screen. Remember that the center of the probe corresponds to the center of the ultrasound screen.

Step 4: Needle insertion and fluid aspiration

- Ensure that there are no surrounding bowel or other organs along the trajectory of the needle.
- Visualize hyperechoic needle tip (in either the in-plane or out-of plane technique) entering the peritoneal cavity (*).

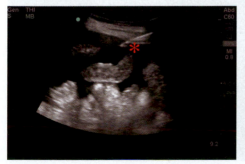
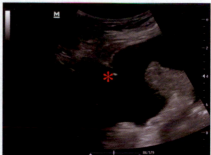

BLADDER VOLUME MEASUREMENT AND ASPIRATION

INDICATIONS

- Measure bladder volume
- Identify the best location for suprapubic aspiration

EQUIPMENT

- Curvilinear probe
- Sterile towels/drape
- Sterile probe cover and gel for dynamic guidance
- Marking pen for static guidance
- Suprapubic supplies

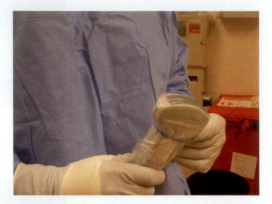

PREPARATION

- Place the patient in the supine position.

STEPS

1. Identify the bladder and measure its volume.
2. Estimate the distance from the skin surface to the bladder.
3. Insert needle and aspirate fluid.

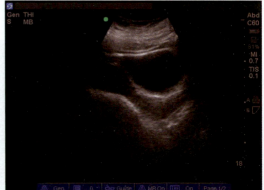

Step 1: Identify the bladder

- Obtain a sagittal view of the bladder by placing the probe in the midline, just above the pubic symphysis.
- The indicator marker on the probe is pointed toward the patient's head. The bladder will appear as a triangular structure filled with anechoic fluid.

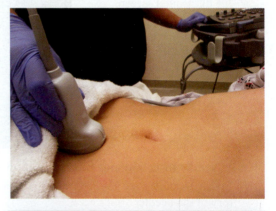

- Obtain a transverse view by placing the probe in the midline, just above the pubic symphysis. The indicator marker on the probe is turned toward the patient's right. The bladder in this cross-section is square shaped.

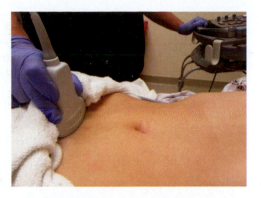

- Determine bladder volume by measuring the bladder in length × width × depth and multiplying by 0.75 to correct for the ellipsoid shape.

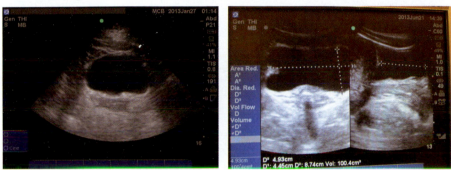

Step 2: Estimate the distance from the skin surface to the bladder

- Orient probe in the transverse plane so that the probe indicator points toward the patient's right.
- Use the markers on the side of the ultrasound screen to estimate the distance from the skin surface to the bladder wall.
- Center the probe so that the maximal diameter of the bladder is in the center of the screen.
- Mark the insertion spot with a sterile marking pen if performing static guidance only.

Step 3: Insert needle and aspirate fluid

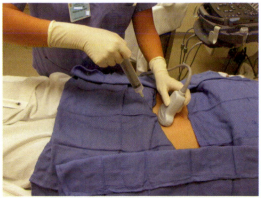

- Position the needle in the center of the probe.
- Advance the probe under dynamic guidance, sliding the probe caudad as the needle is advanced into the bladder to maintain visualization of the needle tip.

SPECIAL CONSIDERATIONS

- Bladder diameters >3.5 cm in the transverse orientation in infants are associated with greater success rates for suprapubic aspiration.
- Empty bladders are often tucked within the pelvis. If the bladder is not easily visualized, angle the probe into the pelvis so that the probe face is angled toward the patient's feet.

16 Pericardiocentesis

Karen S. Cosby

INDICATIONS

- Drain a pericardial effusion resulting in clinical tamponade such as refractory shock or cardiac arrest

IMAGE ACQUISITION AND INTERPRETATION

EQUIPMENT

- 2–5 MHz curvilinear array transducer or a small footprint array transducer
- Marking pen for static approach
- Sterile transducer cover if a dynamic approach is utilized

PREPARATION

- Place patient in supine or semi-recumbent position if possible.
- Ideally, insert a nasogastric tube to empty stomach contents.
- Prepare for sterile procedure. Prepare local anesthetic and agitated saline (shake vigorously immediately prior to administering).

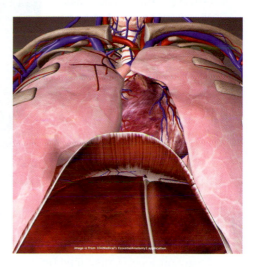

STEPS

1. Identify effusion, evidence of tamponade, and optimal needle entry point.
2. Aspirate effusion under ultrasound guidance.

Step 1: Identify effusion, evidence of tamponade, and optimal needle entry point

- Obtain adequate view of pericardium based on patient body habitus and operator experience.
  - Subxiphoid
  - Parasternal
  - Apical
- Note that pericardial fluid appears as an anechoic space surrounding the heart.
- Confirm presence of a circumferential effusion in at least two views.

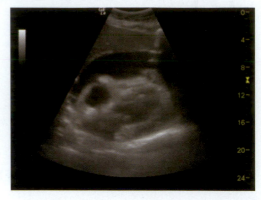

- The optimal needle approach to the pericardium is the site where the effusion is clearly visualized and closest minimizing risk to adjacent structures.

Step 2: Aspirate effusion under ultrasound guidance

- Advance the needle under direct ultrasound visualization into the pericardial space and aspirate.
- Confirm position by injecting and visualizing small amount of agitated saline.

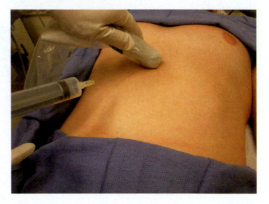

SPECIAL CONSIDERATIONS

- Loculated effusions are difficult to drain with bedside aspiration.
- Distinguish pericardial fluid from pleural effusions.
  - Pericardial fluid will be anterior to the ascending aorta, and should cross the midline.
  - Pleural fluid will be posterior and lateral to the aorta and will not cross the midline.
- Recognize tamponade.
  - Circumferential effusion resulting in right heart diastolic collapse.
  - Refractory shock to cardiac arrest.

17 Thoracentesis

Karen S. Cosby

INDICATIONS

- Identify and measure the size of pleural effusions
- Determine the optimal site for drainage
- Detect loculations or pleural adhesions that may complicate the procedure

IMAGE ACQUISITION AND INTERPRETATION

EQUIPMENT

- A 2.5–5 MHz curvilinear transducer to visualize the lung, pleural space, diaphragm, and liver or spleen, and gives the best overall view
- Marking pen
- Sterile setup for ultrasound probe and procedure

PREPARATION

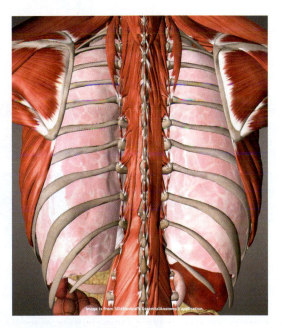

Image is from 3D4Medical's EssentialAnatomy3 application.

- Pre-scan the patient to confirm the size and extent of effusion. A simple effusion will typically be anechoic, free flowing, without loculations, and distant from the lung. A small footprint sector transducer offers an easier view between the ribs.
- Patient positioning for thoracentesis:
  - In the awake patient, sit the patient upright at side of bed, supported by a bedside table or assistant.
  - In the sedated patient, place patient in the lateral decubitus position with back toward the edge of bed and arm positioned out of the field, either raised overhead or across the chest.
- Patient should ideally be able to cooperate to avoid movement during the procedure.

STEPS

1. Evaluate thorax for pleural effusion.
2. Identify landmarks.
3. Mark the site for puncture.
4. Proceed with skin prep, puncture, aspiration, and collection of fluid.
5. After the procedure, rescan for pneumothorax.

Step 1: Evaluate thorax for pleural effusion

- Scan patient in the upright position, first posteriorly between the anterior axillary line and the midline, noting the superior boundary of the fluid. In the recumbent patient, scan over several interspaces, noting the perimeters of the effusion.
- Effusion (*) will usually appear as an anechoic space, but will sometimes have a small amount of internal echoes with fibrinous material that moves with the respiratory cycle.
- Note the distance from the skin to the pleura to estimate the length of needle needed to enter the pleural space.

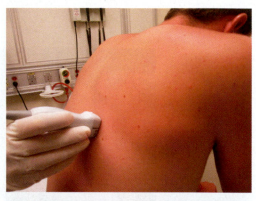

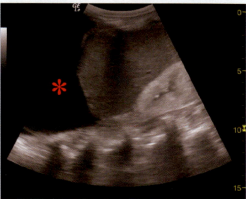

Step 2: Identify landmarks

- Identify the diaphragm and mark its location during the respiratory cycle, noting the most superior border.
- Identify the subdiaphragmatic structures: the liver or spleen.
- Evaluate the presence of lung entering the field during the respiratory cycle. Confirm that at least 10–15 mm of fluid exists between the parietal pleura and lung tissue during the entire respiratory cycle. If not, then abort the procedure.

Step 3: Mark the site for puncture

- Select puncture site.
- Avoid effusions that are loculated. Consider specialty consultation and further imaging prior to intervention.

Step 4: Proceed with skin prep, puncture, aspiration, and collection of fluid following landmarks identified by ultrasound

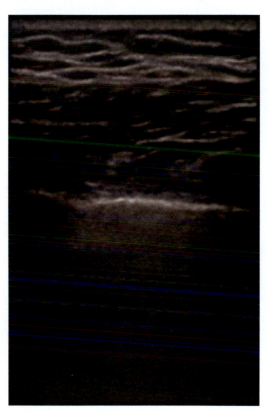

- Perform the aspiration based on landmarks or live if two operators are present.

Step 5: After the procedure, rescan for pneumothorax

SPECIAL CONSIDERATIONS

- Ultrasound guidance optimizes success rate while reducing risk of pneumothorax and inadvertent puncture of adjacent structures (liver, spleen, diaphragm).
- Pediatric/elderly patients may need sedation if they are confused or uncooperative.

18 US-Guided Peripheral Nerve Blocks

Roderick Roxas and Danielle McGee

INDICATIONS

- A safe alternative or adjunct to parenteral narcotics for pain control of injured or painful extremities

IMAGE ACQUISITION AND INTERPRETATION

EQUIPMENT

- High-frequency linear transducer
- Blunt-tipped nerve block needle if available; longer needles for deeper blocks
- Tegaderm
- Povidone-iodine or chlorhexidine swabs
- Local anesthetic
- Short IV tube

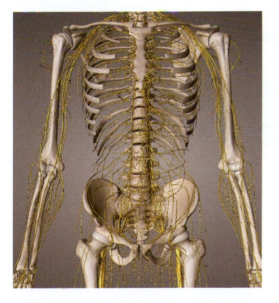

PREPARATION

- Identify relevant anatomy prior to prepping skin and probe for block.
- Prep skin with povidone-iodine or chlorhexidine.
- Prep probe by placing Tegaderm over probe face for added sterility.
- Raise a wheal of local anesthetic at the needle insertion site.
- Extend and externally rotate the arm for distal upper extremity blocks.

ANATOMY

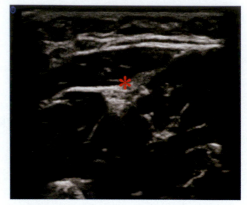

- The hyperechoic perineurium and endoneurium surround the hypoechoic nerve fascicles, creating the classic transverse "honeycomb" appearance of the fascicles (*).
- Nerves are non-compressible and lack color flow with Doppler.

STEPS

1. Visualize the nerve in its desired location.
2. Insert and visualize the needle adjacent to the nerve, then inject anesthetic agent.
3. Confirm achievement of desired block.

ULTRASOUND-GUIDED MEDIAN NERVE BLOCK

STEPS

Step 1: Visualization of the median nerve at the wrist

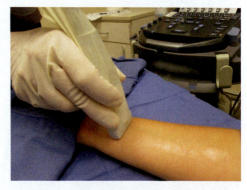

- Scan the wrist in the transverse orientation at the first carpal crease.

Step 2: Insert and visualize the needle adjacent to the nerve, then inject anesthetic agent

- Insert the needle perpendicular to the ultrasound plane. An out-of-plane approach for neural blockade is preferred at this location given the superficial lie of the nerve at the wrist.
- Attach a short IV tube between the needle and the syringe and have an assistant administer the anesthetic under direct visualization.
- Inject anesthetic until the entire nerve is surrounded with anesthetic, typically 5 mL. This may require re-direction of the needle to cover all sides of the median nerve.

ULTRASOUND-GUIDED RADIAL NERVE BLOCK

STEPS

Step 1: Visualization of the radial nerve

- Scan the radial artery from the wrist and move proximally in the transverse orientation. The radial nerve reforms in the mid-forearm lateral to the artery.

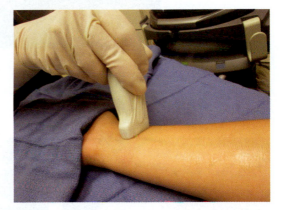

Step 2: Insert and visualize the needle adjacent to the nerve, then inject anesthetic agent

- Insert the needle at a 45-degree angle with respect to the skin, and advance from the radial side of the forearm.
- Advance slowly, in plane, aspirating intermittently to assess for inadvertent vessel puncture.
- Aim for the base of the radial nerve and inject to surround it with anesthetic.
- Readjust the needle trajectory to adequately surround nerve with anesthetic, typically 5 mL.

ULTRASOUND-GUIDED ULNAR NERVE BLOCK

STEPS

Step 1: Visualization of the ulnar nerve in the forearm

- Place probe in the transverse orientation and visualize the ulnar artery (*) at the level of the wrist.

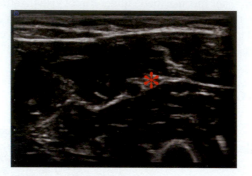

- Trace the artery proximally in the forearm.
- Continue to move proximally and visualize the ulnar nerve (*) in the mid-forearm medial to the artery. The artery deviates from the nerve at this level.

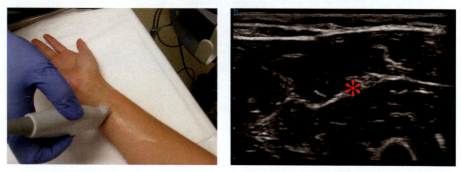

- Note that at this level, anesthesia is provided to both the dorsal and volar sensory branches of the nerve.

Step 2: Insert and visualize the needle adjacent to the nerve and inject anesthetic agent

- Insert needle in an in-plane orientation, very slowly, from the ulnar aspect of the transducer. This allows continuous visualization of the needle along its entire trajectory.

FEMORAL NERVE BLOCK

Steps

Step 1: Visualize the femoral nerve at the inguinal crease

- Align the probe so that it is parallel to the femoral crease.
- Locate femoral artery, an anechoic pulsatile structure adjacent to the femoral vein.
- Locate the iliopsoas muscle, a hypoechoic convex structure lateral and deep to the femoral artery.

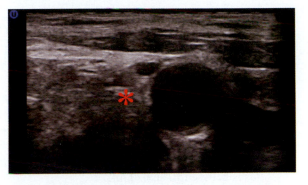

- Locate the femoral nerve, a hyperechoic, bright structure that lies just superficial to the iliopsoas muscle. The fascia iliaca surrounds the femoral nerve.

Step 2: Insert and visualize the needle adjacent to the nerve, then inject anesthetic agent

- Center the femoral nerve on the screen and aim the needle tip medially and parallel to the probe's long axis.
- Visualize the needle tip approaching the femoral nerve.
- Infuse a small amount of anesthetic to confirm needle tip placement. Remember that the needle tip is in the correct location when the fascia iliaca is punctured and the anesthetic surrounds the superficial aspect of the nerve. The needle tip has not yet punctured the fascia iliaca if the anesthetic spreads superficially into the subcutaneous tissues.
- Administer enough anesthetic to cover at least 50% of the femoral nerve's surface area. Typically this is between 10 and 20 mL.

POPLITEAL FOSSA SCIATIC NERVE BLOCK

Preparation

- Place patient in supine position with hip and knee partly flexed.
- Prop up the patient's affected leg with blankets or sheets underneath the calf.

Steps

Step 1: Visualize the sciatic nerve in the popliteal fossa

- Place the transducer in the transverse orientation in the popliteal fossa.
- Locate popliteal artery, an anechoic pulsatile structure under the popliteal vein.

- Scan proximally to visualize the tibial and common peroneal nerve which join to form the sciatic nerve.
- At this level, the biceps femoris muscle is lateral and the semimembranosus muscle is medial to the sciatic nerve.

Step 2: Insert and visualize the needle adjacent to the nerve, then inject anesthetic agent

- Center the sciatic nerve on the screen and aim the needle tip medially and parallel to the probe's long axis.
- Visualize the needle tip approaching the sciatic nerve. Infuse a small amount of anesthetic to confirm needle tip placement.
- Remember that the needle tip is in the correct location when the anesthetic easily surrounds the nerve with further administration.
- Administer enough anesthetic to completely encompass the nerve. Typically this is between 10 and 20 mL.
- Hypoechoic adipose tissue typically surrounds the popliteal sciatic nerve which aids in the nerve's identification.
- Anesthetic must completely surround the nerve to anesthetize both the tibial and common peroneal components.

SPECIAL CONSIDERATIONS

- Regional anesthesia theoretically may mask a clinical compartment syndrome.
- Nerves display less anisotropy than tendons. Additionally, tendons transition into muscles and slide upon digital movement.

19 Lumbar Puncture

John Lemos

INDICATIONS

- Identify non-palpable landmarks in obese patients with BMI >30

IMAGE ACQUISITION AND INTERPRETATION

EQUIPMENT

- High frequency linear probe
- Curvilinear or phased array probe may be used if patient's habitus limits views with the linear probe
- Skin marking pen for static approach
- Lumbar puncture kit

PREPARATION

- Place patient in ideal lumbar puncture (LP) position. This may be in the lateral decubitus or upright position.

STEPS

1. Identify and mark the L4–L5 spinous processes in the transverse (a) and longitudinal (b) orientation.

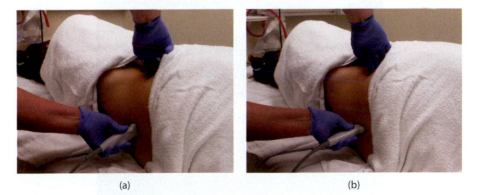

(a)   (b)

2. Mark the associated intervertebral disk space.
3. Proceed with LP using standard procedure.

Step 1: Identify and mark the spinous processes

- Place probe along the mid-lower back at approximately the L4–L5 space.
- Hold the linear probe in longitudinal orientation with indicator directed cephalad.
  - Spinous processes appear as echogenic crescents with posterior shadowing (*).

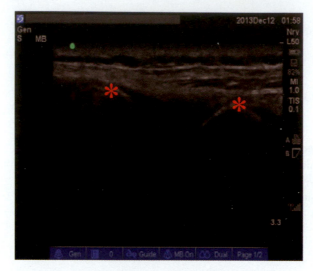

- The processes are separated by the disk space.
- Scan along spinous processes in the transverse orientation to confirm the midline (*).

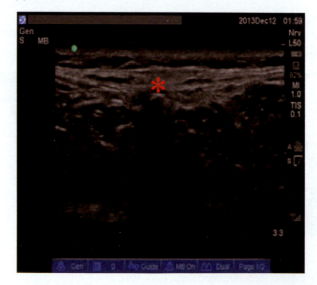

Step 2: Mark the intervertebral disk space between l4–l5

- Utilize the marking pen to clearly define the spinous processes and disk space from both the longitudinal and transverse scanning planes.

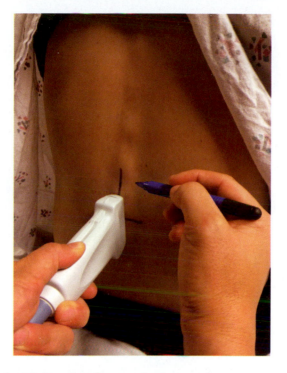

Step 3: Proceed with lP using the standard procedure

SPECIAL CONSIDERATIONS

- A curvilinear probe may also be used if significant subcutaneous tissue limits views with the linear probe.
- Scanning and skin marking is best done prior to establishing a sterile field.
- Patient movement from the position of initial skin marking will alter the ideal location of needle entry—proceed to LP immediately post skin marking. Re-scan if needed.
- The depth of the ligamentum flavum from the skin suggests the need for a longer LP needle pre-procedure.

Further Learning

RECOMMENDED FREE WEB RESOURCES

ACEP SonoGuide http://www.sonoguide.com/introduction.html
Ultrasound Podcast http://www.ultrasoundpodcast.com/

RECOMMENDED ARTICLES

GENERAL

Consensus. ACEP Emergency ultrasound guidelines. *Ann Emerg Med.* 2009;53(4):550–570.
Moore CL, Copel JA. Point-of-care ultrasonography. *N Engl J Med.* 2011;364(8):749–57. doi:10.1056/NEJMra0909487.

TRAUMA

Melniker L, Leibner E, McKenney M, Lopez P, Briggs W, Mancuso C. Randomized controlled clinical trial of point-of-care, limited ultrasonography for trauma in the emergency department: the first sonography outcomes assessment program trial. *Ann Emerg Med.* 2006;48(3):227–235.
Ma OJ, Gaddis G, Norvell JG, Subramanian S. How fast is the focused assessment with sonography for trauma examination learning curve? *Emerg Med Australas.* 2008;20(1):32–37.
Wilkerson RG, Stone MB. Sensitivity of bedside ultrasound and supine anteroposterior chest radiographs for the identification of pneumothorax after blunt trauma. *Acad Emerg Med Off J Soc Acad Emerg Med.* 2010;17(1):11–17. doi:10.1111/j.1553-2712.2009.00628.x.

ECHO AND IVC

Jones AE, Tayal VS, Sullivan DM, Kline JA. Randomized, controlled trial of immediate versus delayed goal-directed ultrasound to identify the cause of nontraumatic hypotension in emergency department patients. *Crit Care Med.* 2004;32(8):1703–1708.
Nagdev AD, Merchant RC, Tirado-Gonzalez A, Sisson CA, Murphy MC. Emergency department bedside ultrasonographic measurement of the caval index for noninvasive determination of low central venous pressure. *YMEM.* 2009:1–6.
Perera P, Mailhot T, Riley D, Mandavia D. The RUSH exam: Rapid Ultrasound in SHock in the evaluation of the critically Ill. *Emerg Med Clin North Am.* 2010;28(1):29–56, vii. doi:10.1016/j.emc.2009.09.010.
Fase AJLMD, Facep VENMD, Fase MBMPHR, et al. Focused cardiac ultrasound in the emergent setting: a consensus statement of the American Society of Echocardiography and American College of Emergency Physicians. *J Am Soc Echocardiogr.* 2010;23(12):1225–1230.
Mantuani D, Nagdev A. Three-view bedside ultrasound to differentiate acute decompensated heart failure from chronic obstructive pulmonary disease. *Am J Emerg Med.* 2013:2012–2014. doi:10.1016/j.ajem.2012.11.028.

LUNG

Lichtenstein DA, Mezière GA. Relevance of lung ultrasound in the diagnosis of acute respiratory failure: the BLUE protocol. *Chest*. 2008;134(1):117–125.

Martindale JL, Noble VE, Liteplo A. Diagnosing pulmonary edema: lung ultrasound versus chest radiography. *Eur J Emerg Med*. 2012;(Im):1–5. doi:10.1097/MEJ.0b013e32835c2b88.

AORTA

Tayal VS, Graf CD, Gibbs MA. Prospective study of accuracy and outcome of emergency ultrasound for abdominal aortic aneurysm over two years. *Acad Emerg Med*. 2003;10(8):867–71.

Hoffmann B, Um P, Bessman ES, Ding R, Kelen GD, McCarthy ML. Routine screening for asymptomatic abdominal aortic aneurysm in high-risk patients is not recommended in emergency departments that are frequently crowded. *Acad Emerg Med Off J Soc Acad Emerg Med*. 2009;16(11):1242–1250. doi:10.1111/j.1553-2712.2009.00502.x.

Hoffmann B, Bessman ES, Um P, Ding R, McCarthy ML. Successful sonographic visualisation of the abdominal aorta differs significantly among a diverse group of credentialed emergency department providers. *Emerg Med J EMJ*. 2010. doi:10.1136/emj.2009.086462.

RENAL

Gaspari RJ, Horst K. Emergency ultrasound and urinalysis in the evaluation of flank pain. *Acad Emerg Med*. 2005;12(12):1180–4. doi:10.1197/j.aem.2005.06.023.

Herbst MK, Rosenberg G, Daniels B, et al. Effect of provider experience on clinician-performed ultrasonography for hydronephrosis in patients with suspected renal colic. *Ann Emerg Med*. 2014. doi:10.1016/j.annemergmed.2014.01.012.

Moore CL, Bomann S, Daniels B, et al. Derivation and validation of a clinical prediction rule for uncomplicated ureteral stone—the STONE score: retrospective and prospective observational cohort studies. *BMJ*. 2014;348(mar26 2):g2191–g2191. doi:10.1136/bmj.g2191.

BILIARY

Summers SM, Scruggs W, Menchine MD, et al. A prospective evaluation of emergency department bedside ultrasonography for the detection of acute cholecystitis. *Ann Emerg Med*. 2010;56(2):114–122.

Jang TB, Ruggeri W, Dyne P, Kaji AH. The learning curve of resident physicians using emergency ultrasonography for cholelithiasis and cholecystitis. *Acad Emerg Med*. 2010;17(11):1247–1252.

FIRST TRIMESTER

Moore C, Todd WM, O'Brien E, Lin H. Free fluid in Morison's pouch on bedside ultrasound predicts need for operative intervention in suspected ectopic pregnancy. *Acad Emerg Med*. 2007;14(8):755–758.

Jang T, Ruggeri W, Dyne P, Kaji A. Learning curve of emergency physicians using emergency bedside sonography for symptomatic first-trimester pregnancy. *J Ultrasound Med*. 2010;29(10):1423.

Bloch AJ, Bloch SA, Lyon M. Correlation of β-human chorionic gonadotropin with ultrasound diagnosis of ectopic pregnancy in the ED. *Am J Emerg Med*. 2013;31(5):876–7. doi:10.1016/j.ajem.2013.01.009.

Appendix

Fox JC, Solley M, Anderson CL, Zlidenny A, Lahham S, Maasumi K. Prospective evaluation of emergency physician performed bedside ultrasound to detect acute appendicitis. *Eur J Emerg Med*. 2008;15(2):80–5. doi:10.1097/MEJ.0b013e328270361a.
Santillanes G, Simms S, Gausche-Hill M, et al. Prospective evaluation of a clinical practice guideline for diagnosis of appendicitis in children. *Acad Emerg Med*. 2012. doi:10.1111/j.1553-2712.2012.01402.x.

Ocular

Blaivas M. Bedside emergency department ultrasonography in the evaluation of ocular pathology. *Acad Emerg Med*. 2000;7(8):947–50.
Yoonessi R, Hussain A, Jang TB. Bedside ocular ultrasound for the detection of retinal detachment in the emergency department. *Acad Emerg Med*. 2010;17(9):913–917.

Soft Tissue

Tayal VS, Hasan N, Norton HJ, Tomaszewski CA. The effect of soft-tissue ultrasound on the management of cellulitis in the emergency department. *Acad Emerg Med*. 2006;13(4):384–388.
Gaspari RJ, Resop D, Mendoza M, Kang T, Blehar D. A Randomized controlled trial of incision and drainage versus ultrasonographically guided needle aspiration for skin abscesses and the effect of methicillin-resistant Staphylococcus aureus. *Ann Emerg Med*. 2011;57(5):483–491.e1.
Srikar, A BM. Sonography first for subcutaneous abscess and cellulitis evaluation. *J Ultrasound Med*. 2012:1509–1512.

MSK

Stone MB, Wang R, Price DD. Ultrasound-guided supraclavicular brachial plexus nerve block vs procedural sedation for the treatment of upper extremity emergencies. *Am J Emerg Med*. 2008;26(6):706–710.
Vieira RL, Levy JA. Bedside ultrasonography to identify hip effusions in pediatric patients. *Ann Emerg Med*. 2009.

DVT

Kline JA, O'Malley PM, Tayal VS, Snead GR, Mitchell AM. Emergency clinician-performed compression ultrasonography for deep venous thrombosis of the lower extremity. *Ann Emerg Med*. 2008;52(4):437–445. doi:10.1016/j.annemergmed.2008.05.023.
Crisp JG, Lovato LM, Jang TB. Compression ultrasonography of the lower extremity with portable vascular ultrasonography can accurately detect deep venous thrombosis in the emergency department. *Ann Emerg Med*. 2010;56(6):601–610.

Peds

Riera A, Hsiao AL, Langhan ML, Goodman TR, Chen L. Diagnosis of intussusception by physician novice sonographers in the emergency department. *Ann Emerg Med.* 2012;60(3):264–268. doi:10.1016/j.annemergmed.2012.02.007.

Shah VP, Tunik MG, Tsung JW. Prospective evaluation of point-of-care ultrasonography for the diagnosis of pneumonia in children and young adults. *JAMA Pediatr.* 2013;167(2): 1–7. doi:10.1001/2013.jamapediatrics.107

Procedures

Tirado A, Nagdev A, Henningsen C, Breckon P, Chiles K. Ultrasound-guided procedures in the emergency department-needle guidance and localization. *Emerg Med Clin North Am.* 2013;31(1):87–115. doi:10.1016/j.emc.2012.09.008.

Tirado A, Wu T, Noble VE, et al. Ultrasound-guided procedures in the emergency department-diagnostic and therapeutic asset. *Emerg Med Clin North Am.* 2013;31(1):117–49. doi:10.1016/j.emc.2012.09.009.

Index